Charles R. Broadbent

A medical treatise on the causes and curability of consumption,

laryngitis,

Chronic catarrh and diseases of the air-passages : combining the treatment by

inhalation of medicated vapors : also, a new and accurate method for the diagnosis

of consumptio

Charles R. Broadbent

A medical treatise on the causes and curability of consumption, laryngitis,
Chronic catarrh and diseases of the air-passages : combining the treatment by inhalation of medicated vapors : also, a new and accurate method for the diagnosis of consumptio

ISBN/EAN: 9783337730277

Printed in Europe, USA, Canada, Australia, Japan

Cover: Foto ©ninafisch / pixelio.de

More available books at **www.hansebooks.com**

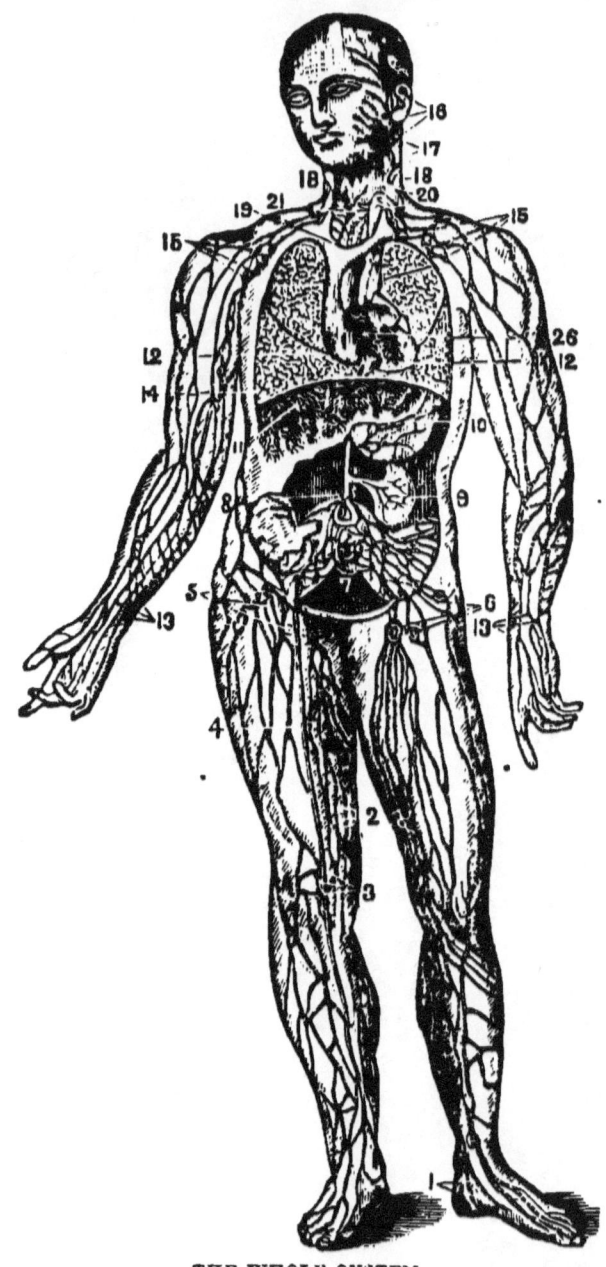

THE WHOLE SYSTEM.

15, The Lungs. 26, The Heart. 11, The Liver. 10, The Stomach. 5, 6, 8, 9, The Intestines. 7, The Bladder.

A MEDICAL TREATISE

ON THE CAUSES AND CURABILITY OF

CONSUMPTION,

LARYNGITIS, CHRONIC CATARRH, AND DISEASES OF THE AIR-PASSAGES.

COMBINING THE TREATMENT BY INHALATION OF MEDICATED VAPORS.

ALSO, A NEW AND ACCURATE METHOD FOR THE

DIAGNOSIS OF CONSUMPTION;

OR, HOW TO DETECT ITS SIGNS AND SYMPTOMS IN ITS VARIOUS STAGES.

ALSO,

INCLUDING MANY CHRONIC AND NERVOUS DISEASES, HUMORS, FITS, &c. WITH AN APPENDIX ON TOBACCO, Showing its injurious effects on both body and mind; PHRENOLOGY AND MESMERISM.

BY CHARLES R. BROADBENT, M. D.

BOSTON:
DAMRELL & WELCH, PRINTERS, 22 COURT STREET.
1862.

INTRODUCTION.

I now present to the public my new work, which is A Treatise on the Causes and Curability of Tubercular and Bronchial Consumption, Laryngitis, Chronic Catarrh, and Diseases of the Air-Passages, Health, &c.; combining the Treatment by Inhalation of Medicated Vapors, designed both for the student of medicine as well as the general reader. I at first intended to issue a larger work, but, upon more mature reflection, I deemed it best to publish it in its present form and size. The price of a work as large and costly as I at first contemplated, would have restricted the sale considerably, in placing it beyond the reach of those in limited circumstances. These objections, together with the great labor and cost, and also want of time to prepare such a work, have induced me thus to issue it; and I think it preferable, taking everything into consideration. I have labored to be brief, perspicuous and comprehensive, and at the same time, to give clear and full description of the different subjects, so that I might impart instruction.

The reader will perceive that I have tried to adapt this treatise to the capacity of the popular reader, as well as the student of medicine. We must depend for patronage for a work of this kind upon all classes of the community; and indeed the success of our reformatory course in medicine, depends much upon disseminating among them correct views on these subjects, which shows obviously the utility and importance of such a work. All classes are daily suffering from the want of more information on the laws which govern their organization, and which are constantly being violated through ignorance.

This fact ought to convince every one that there is a necessity of studying those laws, both to prevent and cure disease.

Great truths are taught, which, if fully understood, implicitly believed, and judiciously followed, would lead to an almost total annihilation of Pulmonary Consumption.

The author has had an opportunity of addressing about fifty thousand persons in the principal cities of New England, where he has given lectures for twelve years, on Physiology, Health, &c.,—and thus of personally presenting and enforcing his views by direct examples, and prompt, practical results and demonstrations.

In 1845 he discovered his mode of treatment by Inhalation; and, knowing the uses of the Lungs, he thereby laid the foundation of a scientific, rational, and certain method of elucidating and treating their diseases.

For eighteen years, diseases of the chest have been his study. To notice the effects of climate as a curative or preventative agent, he has visited many of the States of the American Union, England, and some parts even of Europe, — seeking for knowledge and light on the diseases of the Lungs; making himself everywhere as fully acquainted as possible with the peculiarities of each locality, both in the nature and prevalence of Consumption, and the peculiar methods adopted for its prevention and cure by some of the first physicians in Europe and America.

In conclusion, he would say, that, in presenting this work to the public, and to consumptive invalids, he makes no apologies, or statements of what wonders he can perform; but simply presents facts, which he asks all to thoroughly read, and examine for themselves.

C. R. BROADBENT, M. D.

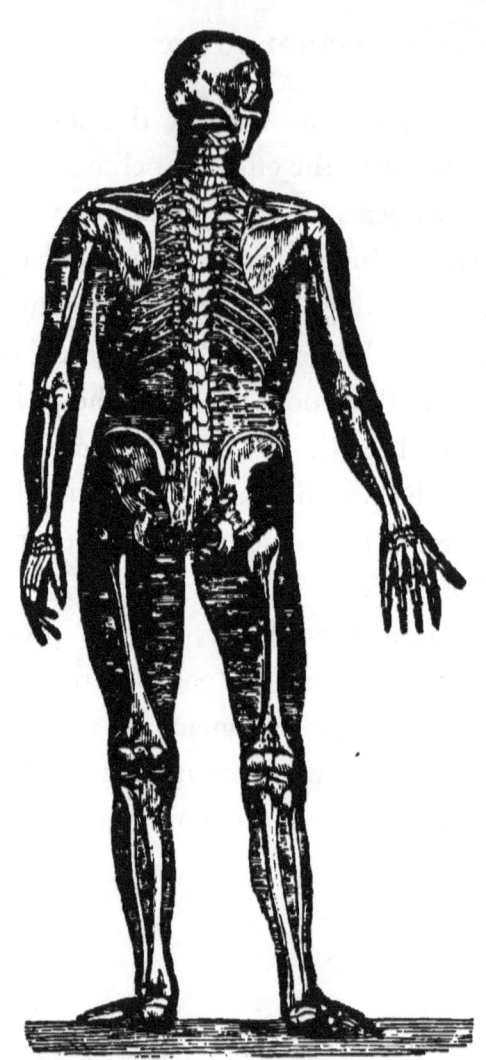

BACK VIEW OF A SKELETON.

CONSUMPTION:

ITS CAUSES AND CURABILITY.

The importance of an inquiry into the causes, and correct information as to the curability of Pulmonary Consumption, cannot be over-estimated, especially when we consider the very general prevalence of this disease and the amount of mortality it occasions.

There is no country in the known world where Consumption and its kindred affections, immediately connected with the thoracic organs,—laryngitis, inflammation and ulceration of the mucous follicles of the throat, bronchitis, &c.,—are so common as in the United States.

From fifty to sixty thousand persons of all ages, from childhood to advanced age, are annually extinguished by this scourge alone. More hearts are caused to bleed, and the happiness of families blasted more by the severing of the dearest ties of life by this destroyer, than by any other disease in the whole catalogue of medical nosology. Besides this, what becomes more melancholy, Consumption selects its victims, not, like some other diseases, from the extremes of life, but from those who are in the pride of youth, or in the prime and vigor of life. Although this statement, as far as past general statistics are concerned, is correct, it will now admit of many and every-day exceptions, since the modes of living, especially in American cities, have become so artificial that children of tender years are daily becoming its victims in some one of its Protean forms,—scrofula, manifested by enlarged tonsillary glands, hip-joint and spinal irritations, which all belong to the one great class, and proceed from the same cause; impure state of the blood, from confined and vitiated air; bad and insufficient food; improper clothing and habits of dress; and insufficient exercise in the open air.

The profession, as well as the community, have been so strongly impressed with the belief that the disease is necessarily fatal, that any one who would have maintained the opposite opinion, would, until within a very short period of time, have been looked upon only in the light of a boasting pretender. So strongly was this opinion, inherited from our ancestors, impressed upon the minds of the faculty, that their general decided opinion, in cases of symptoms that assumed the consumptive character only, has resulted in the premature death of thousands, by an abandonment of all timely and proper aid; and, at the same time, this phantom of prejudice or ignorance served as a stumbling-block in the way of scientific inquiry into the true pathology of Consumption, which, by the energetic efforts of a few meritorious physicians, has demonstrated the fact that Consumption is as curable as other diseases.

The great obstacle to the true progress of medical inquiry, and the developement of skill in curing this intricate and complicated class of maladies, has been a professional oligarchy. A combination of a clique, who were too often supported in their power by the secret springs of wealth, and by certain established rules of government and etiquette for their own self-acquiring power or patronage, have dared to pronounce a wholesale condemnation of irregularity upon every one, or class even, who had the courage to conscientiously advocate views at variance with their received theories and aristocratical regulations, in order thereby to bring every one into disrepute that dared to differ from them. This system of professional government, which originated in the European schools, has assumed to execute the same conservative notions by the leaders in America, as though the human mind could be hindered from investigation, and thought fettered or crushed by human enactments or dogmas of faith, especially when the necessity of such enquiry has its foundation in benevolence and duty to suffering humanity. To such an unwise extent has this prejudice of professional cliquism been carried in the United States, even to the great injury of the suffering of the community, who can have no interest in professional dogmas, that the most successful and enlightened practitioners in this special clas of complaints are found without the pale of the caste, and are arrayed as so many mountebanks. Precisely under such opposition and persecution has every great discovery in the world of science been made, and triumphed. Indeed it seems necessary for the progress and development of truth for it to meet not only with opposition, but oppression. The masses of mankind will think and reason and inquire for themselves, in spite of human enactments or the rigid rules of conservative bodies.

Appropriately applying this reasoning to the practical investigations into the causes and nature of tuberculosis and bronchial consumption, pathological investigations have shown, in the clearest manner, that recovery from this disease often does take place, even in many instances where large caverns were found in the lungs, from the softening or ulceration and discharge of the tubercular matter by expectoration; and, ever since the able investigations of Laennec, modern pathologists have been diligent in accumulating and substantially proving the correctness of his views and statements.

The brilliant light shed upon or steps by the knowledge of *auscultation* and *percussion* enables us to separate those diseases from Consumption which were formerly so often confounded with it (and daily now are by those physicians who do not avail themselves of the only true guides of this science), and trace the successive steps of recovery in our patients. Sir James Clark, physician to Queen Victoria, remarks that pathological anatomy has perhaps never afforded more conclusive evidence in proof of the curability of a disease than it has in that of Tubercular Consumption. Dr. J. Hughes Bennett, one of the ablest and most brilliant pathologists of the present day, says that during five years of his acting in that capacity to the Royal Infirmary of Edinburgh, during which period he performed and recorded the results of two thousand cases, one great fact became impressed upon his mind,—that in no organic disease were appearances to be found, as in the lungs, indicating a spontaneous cure by nature; and he gives his decided opinion, drawn from experience, of the perfect curability of Pulmonary Consumption.

Drs. Forbes, Louis, and Trumbull, of the Hospital for Consumptives, of Liverpool, and many other able physicians, both in Europe and America, now all concur in the curability of Consumption.

For my own part, I know Consumption to be curable; for I have often cured it, in hundreds of instances, and in cases where patients had had abcesses and caverns in the lungs of three years' standing. No one need despair of a cure. If he seeks timely aid and follows my directions as to the mode of treatment, his hopes will be realized with crowning success.

Tubercular Depositions are not, however, peculiar to the lungs. They are found in the bowels and other glandular parts of the body, and not unfrequently in the brain itself. In those cases denominated Bronchial Consumption, the deposition first takes place in the delicate mucous membrane back of the throat, the larynx, and the glands that line the throat, extending down to the branches of the trachea or windpipe, and so into the innumerable branches of air-tubes, which alone can properly be called Bronchitis; and when left alone the chronic inflammation invariably terminates in ulceration or disorganization, and death.

The complications of Throat and Chest affections conclusively proves the necessity of a nice discrimination in their character, by auscultation and other scientific modes of examination, before the basis of a successful treatment can be laid or hoped for.

In a large majority of instances, the foundation for Consumption is laid in childhood and early life,—among the causes of which may be recorded the constant inhalation of bad or impure air; unwholesome and insufficient food; the use of confectionery and pastries; keeping the temperature of the body, particularly the extremities, too low, from a deficiency of clothing; sedentary habits; improper or late hours; and often, in the youth of both sexes, wasting habits silently acquired, which insidiously enervates the vital energies. The continued operation of these causes engenders that state of the blood spoken of. Debilitating excesses of all kinds are sufficient, in some of the most healthy, to cause Consumption, especially in the youth of both sexes.

As an evidence of the injurious effects of breathing damp and unwholesome air, and its agencies in the cause of scrofula and tubercles, it is worthy of notice that tubercles may be produced at will in some of the the lower animals, by confining them in damp places, and feeding them with unwholesome food. This was done with rabbits, by Drs. Barron, Jenner, and Carswell. It is a fact that cows, long confined, without exercise, in dark or unhealthy sheds or stalls, die tuberculous.

What, then, are the general indications for the cure of Consumption? It has been clearly shown that it is not merely a disease of the lungs, but a constitutional condition also, in which there is debility, an impaired digestion and assimilation, so that the blood, which should nourish every part, becomes impure, and is rendered insufficient to nourish and build up the lungs. We have, therefore, in treating this disease, not merely to prevent the local state of irritation or inflammation, or tuberculization, from resulting in disorganization, but to cleanse the blood, and restore the energies of the stomach and digestive organs; so that a healthy state of the whole system may be produced, and the necessary principals imparted to the blood, through the only natural channel—the chyle, and the performance of the healthy functions of assimilation effected,—by which means we can prevent the further formation of tubercles, and remove those already formed by the process of absorption.

The important plan of treatment adopted by the author, which has been so successful in his hands in curing Pulmonary Consumption, is, in the first place, to restore the stomach and assimilative functions to a healthy, normal condition. This is done by a judicious and very discriminate use of a course of the mildest tonic and alterative vegetable agents, made most acceptable to the patient by a studied scientific attention to their preparation. The apetite becomes invigorated, and regulated to a healthy demand, and a relish is by this means produced for the food not before possessed; so that the patient instinctively looks to these auxiliary agents as a necessary part of his dietetics.

This end being obtained, the most nutritious articles of animal food can be borne, such as beef and pork steaks, mutton chops, soft boiled eggs, custards, oysters, good milk cream, and all the most nutritive and digestive articles of animal food, so important to produce good blood, and raise the healing powers of nature, that she may send the restorative energies to every minute part of the vital organs.

How widely different this tonic and nutritive course,

the result of modern and scientific observation, when contrasted with that debilitating routine system of drugging with calomel, antimony, jalap, ipecac, and squills, formerly, and even now, often pursued by some physicians, whose energies are insufficient to their emergencies, and who look discouragingly on, and see patients die by the thousand of a malady every way curable! Well may the consumptive take courage, well may his hope revive, at the assurance that we live in an age of progress and improvement!

To fulfill other very important indications, and which are looked upon by the author as vitally indispensable to the success of treatment, is the regulations of the secretions; and the chief are those of the lungs themselves, the liver, skin, and kidneys. We have seen that the digestive organs are the inlet by which imperfectly elaborated particles obtain access to the blood; and these, the lungs, liver, skin, and kidneys, are the excreting organs, by the healthful activity of which they should be expelled.

When we consider the fact that the lungs have a surface of twenty-four hundred cubic feet, provided by nature to disengage carbonic acid gas, in the shape of vapor, from the blood,—which is gathered by three gallons of blood passing through the lungs every three minutes for the purpose, after having carried the revivifying agent, oxygen, to every part of the body, and

2*

then, returning, throw off this carbon and receive more oxygen,— how vitally important to every consumptive patient, and to every person, that they inhale the purest air both day and night, that this healthy and necessary secretion of the lungs shall be kept up! and how necessary to obtain this information from one who devotes the energies of his life to develop such important facts! The liver, too, which is the largest secretory gland in the body, performs a wonderful function. In the majority of cases of consumptive diseases it is much deranged, and often is the primary seat of future disease to the lungs, through the nerves, and medium of sympathy to the stomach, duodenum, and to the pancreas, and so to the diaphragm, and so in turn to the lungs; causing the phenomena of Dyspeptic Consumption. Thousands of fatal cases are truly Dyspeptic Consumption, and have their first starting-point from the liver and digestive organs being deranged ; and, until the healthy function of the liver is restored, the lungs are made to do a double duty for both, which accounts for its implication of irritation in various ways.

Every person is aware, from the amount of secretion daily carried off by the bladder, what an immense labor the kidneys have to perform ; but few, however, of the popular readers who are not versed in physiology, can conceive how constantly dependent are our lives upon the perfect integrity of these organs ; for, were they to fail in maintaining the necessary secretion of this allotted function, a few hours alone often would be sufficient to produce death, by the fact of the deleterious particles being carried again into the blood, poisoning the brain, and terminating in coma and death. It is but a year since a lady well known to us was travelling, in the care of a gentleman, in a stage coach, and, through diffidence or modesty, neglected for a length of time to attend to the demands of nature upon the bladder, until the mischief was so great that death, with untold agony was the consequence. And it is but a short time since another fatal instance, somewhat similar, came to our knowledge. A lady in pregnancy suffered the gravid uterus to press long upon the neck of the bladder, producing such retention of the urine, that, the poisonous properties of urea being retained in the blood so long, the case terminated fatally, from a neglect to obtain relief in season,—just from undue modesty, or false delicacy in asking medical assistance.

The patient will then take into consideration, with us, the momentous importance of attending to the healthy state of the kidneys in treating consumptive diseases; and the gratitude that should be felt towards one who will step out of the pale of conservatism to enlighten the community in regard to those organs, upon the healthy condition of which depends not only health but life itself, I need not stop here to consider.

The function of the skin is not of minor importance to that of the kidneys, or of other organs mentioned, in taking out a wonderful amount of worn out and effete matter from the system. But, as it would swell the pages of this popular treatise too full to go into a lengthy dissertation of its merits, and the necessity of sustaining its due healthy action, we must explain the matter to our patients personally or by letter.

SYMPTOMS OF CONSUMPTION.

This disease often commences so very insidiously, especially in girls and females who have grown rapidly, that it is permitted to advance very far before the case is brought to the observation of the physician,—a circumstance much to be regetted. Advice from the best source, from one who has made the causes and curability of lung diseases his special study and inquiry, should be obtained as early as any unfavorable symptoms are manifested. Cough is one of the early symptoms, usually coming on slowly, at first very slight, occurring in the morning or in making any unusual exertion, as going up stairs, &c.

Oppression at the chest is a common symptom, accompanied with pain at the top of the lungs, or under the collar bones and under the shoulder blades. Pallor of the countenance; a bluish and settled appearance under the eyes; coldness of the feet and hands; a morbid and capricious appetite; languor and debility; and great disinclination to active exertion, either bodily or mental, — should warn the individual or friends that some mischief is brewing, and of the necessity of help. Now the palms of the hands and soles of the feet begin to feel dry at one period of the day, with a feverish spell at night, either preceeded or followed with perspiration and chill. Sound sleep is hardly obtained. Expectoration comes on in the second stage of the disease; and diarrhœa, alternating frequently with constipation of the bowels, swelling of the feet and ankles, dryness of the lips, and cankerous sores of the mouth, mark the third stage of consumption,— also frequent expectoration or spitting of blood.

Shortness of breath, pain in the chest, hectic fever, combined with night sweats and chills, are among the leading symptoms of approaching Consumption. Hoarseness of the voice, dryness of the throat and air-passages, a disposition to "hem," and irritation about the larynx, and soreness of the upper part of the chest, are the frequent symptoms and attendants of Bronchial Consumption.

The menstrual function in many females becomes suppressed during the earlier stages of Consumption, and in others the disease advances far towards its termination without this function being interrupted.

When skillful advice is not early sought, it is rarely attributed to a correct cause, and irreparable injury is often produced to the constitution by the patient taking heating and driving medicines, which, instead of effecting its establishment, drives the blood unduly to the lungs, producing congestion, and setting up the commencement of inflammation, and consequently ulceration.

Strictly connected with this subject of periodical derangement, as indicating a strong consumptive disposition, is a well known and marked habit of some females, especially at certain periods ⬤life,—puberty—called chlorosis. The countenance puts on a peculiar sallow or greenish appearance, the space immediately below the eyes appears dark or purple, the apetite is morbid or fastidious, the patient is troubled with frightful dreams or disturbed sleep, great coldness of the extremities, the nervous system becomes morbidly sensitive or irritable, and great languor or inability to physical exertion is manifested. The whole cause of morbid sympathies in this case proceeds from an impure and unhealthy state of the blood, and should excite the utmost apprehension for the integrity of the lungs before a favorable opportunity of cure passes. This class of female patients often meets with the inroads of Consumption, as a sympathetic irritation, long continued from a local inflammation and morbid irritability of the nerves of the uterus and reproductive organs. In this class of cases, involving sympathetic or irritative Consumption, the treatment must be especially directed to the restoration of the integrity of those organs which play so conspicuous a part in the economy of health, and to insure the future prospects of a healthy conception, without entailing misery upon offspring, by transmitting a permanent predisposition to constitutional Consumption.

The complications of Consumption are numerous:— asthma; whooping-cough; chronic and acute affections of the pleura; dropsy, or water in the chest; diseases of the heart, involving thickening of the valves, or enlargement; palpitation; suffocating sense of feeling on going up a hill or ascending a flight of stairs, and a sense of constriction. Chronic diarrhœa or dysentery are also among the complications of Consumption. Among these asthma, difficulty of breathing, palpitation, and diarrhœa should require the earliest attention,

Marasmus, or a wasting habit in children, is Consumption arising from a scrofulous or an impure state of the blood, caused by bad and insufficient clothing, want of exercise in the open air, &c.; and should excite the most serious apprehension on the part of parents to have the causes and the condition of the system spedily removed, or else fatal Consumption will be the consequence.

Many of the most fatal and melancholy instances of

Bronchial Consumption are daily brought to the notice of the observant physician, originating in a neglect to attend to slight colds or catarrh. This, at first, is only confined to the mucous membrane of the *nose and frontal sinus*. A profuse secretion is the consequence of the inflammatory action locally set up in the mucous glands, —it is neglected; the patient thinks it will wear off, using his own judgement; it silently but gradually extends its influence of irritation downwards; it passes the epiglottis of the larynx, and enters the lungs and larger bronchi; and then commences a renewed irritation, when new and more troublesome symptoms begin to be manifested. In this stage of the case, it comes to the notice of the physician.

Just so long as people will more willingly pay their money for the gratification of their vision, and the various scenes of pleasure, or for dissipation and enervating luxuries, than to be informed in regard to the laws of health and life, regarding the true conservator of human health as a mercenary agent, just so long will the causes be in operation which induce this disease and its melancholy results. It is this last class of maladies, confined to the mucous membrane and glands that line the air-passages, that I have been very successful in treating, by the administration of Medicated Vapors by Inhalation. Very many cases that had been pronounced as incurable tubercular phthisis by the old school faculty, where loss of voice, hoarseness, and expectoration of blood have been the long-attendant symptoms, I have succeeded in restoring to perfect health; and the patients ultimately recovered their natural voice.

The soothing and quieting effects of these Vapors is brought immediately to act upon the parts locally irritated and diseased, by the gentle inhalation of the vapor from a bottle arranged expressly for the purpose, and is used by the patient without the aid of the physician, in his own room, several times a day, according to the urgency of the case. By bringing the treatment immediately within the hands of the patient in such a soothing manner, hope is revived, much expense from the daily visits of the physician is saved, and the stomach is not taxed with medicines. So successful has this mode of treatment been in my hands, which I had the honor of introducing in New England nearly eighteen years since, that I believe, if seasonable treatment was adopted, ninety-nine cases in the hundred could be cured perfectly. In Tubercular Consumption, it is already working wonders, in the ready mode of carrying its healing, stimulating, and restorative action to every minute air-cell and branch of the air-tubes; almost instantly putting a stop to the cough, relieving pain, calming irritation, arousing the malignant and ulcerated cavities to put on a healing process, and stimulating the absorbents to take out of the lungs the tubercular deposits.

It is a matter of great question in my mind if agents in the form of vapor alone will cure Pulmonary Tuberculosis from an hereditary cause, without the aid of nutrition and tonics, carried into the blood through the medium of the assimilative functions, to correct a scrofulous or bad state of the blood, the constitutional condition of which is the cause of deposition of tubercles in the lungs. But the inhalation of these medicated vapors are a powerful auxiliary means even in this form of Consumption.

PRACTICAL OBSERVATIONS

ON THE

CAUSES AND CURABILITY OF TUBERCULAR AND BRONCHIAL CONSUMPTION.

The plan of treatment so successfully instituted and administered by the author is Medicated Vapors, carried to the lungs and the seat of disease by breathing, or inhaling, in an easy, gentle, and soothing manner. By this direct method, the virtues of the most benign and healing medicinal agents are so happily prepared and developed to such a perfect system, by the past experience of many years, as to be made to traverse every air-cell and tube of the lungs speedily and readily, without the very uncertain and indirect course of putting the drugs into the stomach, where the disease is not. Every intelligent person, having any knowledge of the anatomy of the respiratory organs, must see that putting drugs into the stomach cannot reach the lungs, unless in a most indirect manner, through the medium of the circulation, which is so uncertain that weeks must be required to accomplish what can be done in a few minutes by inhalation.

The lungs and organs of respiration are entirely

separated from the stomach and digestive organs by a partition, and a separate passage conveys air to the lungs, beside the one that conveys food to the stomach. Let it be distinctly kept in memory, that not one well-marked case of Tubercular Consumption can be produced, cured by putting medicines in the stomach, while very many can be by the author's system of inhalation. The human stomach was designed for food and nutriment only, for building up and sustaining the waste of the body, from the devastation of oxygen, or chemical action, so that the vital forces should at all times predominate and maintain the ascendency, otherwise dissolution would be the inevitable result.

Let us consider what is the effect of putting drugs into the stomach:— Is it not nausea, sickness, loss of appetite, vomiting, and consequent debility? Doctors, for hundreds, thousands of years, have told you to take medicine to strengthen the system, and the mass of the community, who never think for themselves, take it for granted it is so, their credulity captivated by the marvellous secrecy of nostrums. Thus the world has reasoned, or rather acted from adoption, until the whole race have become so degenerate from the preposterous system of drugging with the most deadly poisons that a fearful consideration presents itself, whether the ability of propagation shall be continued; such is the sad effeminacy.

Look at the poor distressed mortals that you see around you on every side, in every house, and in every street; the pale, faded and wan countenances, the shrunken muscles and withered features, all show forth a most melancholy truth, that they are the sad and more melancholy victims of some painful system of drug poisoning, either in their own person or in their immediate progenitors. For the sins of the fathers are visited upon their children, even to the third and fourth generations. Look at your children, afflicted with catarrh, scrofula, enlarged tonsils, and swelled glands, ulcerated throats, bronchitis, and that most distressing of all disorders, acute laryngitis, or membranous croup; these, with dropsical effusions, either of the brain or chest, and a general emaciation, are all the results of a long series of drug medication and poisoning, combined with the concomitants of the luxuries of modern life; a multiform, complex system of artful, suicidal destruction of human life, so melancholy in its nature, that when duly brought home to our reflection, is sufficient to cause humanity to shudder and stand aghast.

Is it not time to look about you? Behold your young children, the victims of spinal curvatures, hip-joint diseases, scrofula, and pulmonary tubercular consumption. Look at your daughters, fading and going down to a premature grave, just at the age when they should be developing into mature physical strength! Why is our race shortened down to thirty-three years, instead of three score and ten? Why do we die as suicides, so that not one natural death takes place in five hundred. This is an appaling fact which cannot be controverted. Is there no cause for all this? Is there not an awful responsibility resting upon you to know yourselves, and understand the laws of your physical being? Returning to the all-important consideration of our subject, can you not perceive that mercury, calomel, antimony, arsenic, and other deadly mineral poisons, now used by the old school physicians, and which have been used for centuries, have come down to us as the barbarous relics of the darker ages of the world, were never intended by our Maker to be put into the human stomach? They form no part of the elementary materials of our bodies. The human stomach was designed for the reception of pure, healthy food, and nutrition only.

If you wish for a practical demonstration that there is no such thing as strength or nourishment in drugs, as you are told there is, abstain from eating and taking nourishment for a few weeks; take calomel, and jalap, and antimony, and instead of being sustained and sustaining the full image of our Maker, we shall become emaciated, but the wreck of matter, and a shadow of what we once were, a fit subject for the undertaker.

Dear reader, fathers and parents, throw " physic to the dogs," and provide for yourselves, your children, and families, good and healthy food; live consistently with the laws of life and health — laws which certainly govern your being — or, if ye violate, ye must certainly pay the penalty in sickness and premature death.

Know, then, that it is your duty to study yourselves, and recognize your responsibility to your Maker. Live consistently, and sickness will be banished; the goddess of health will once more return to greet you, to cheer your domestic circle, your homes and firesides; youth will smile in perpetual virginity, and your end shall be sweet and as gentle as the last flickerings of an expiring taper.

Continue to violate those laws, and your now happy homes will be saddened by the couch of sickness; and though it may be hidden beneath the display of fashion and pride, come it will, in the form of that Messenger that seals the fate of thousands of our beloved daughters, and annually extinguishes the lights of sixty thousand of our fellow-beings in the United States every year.

> "With step as noiseless as the summer airs,
> Who comes in beautiful decay — her eyes
> Dissolving with a feverish glow of light;
> And on her cheek a rosy tint, as if the tip
> Of beauty's finger pressed it there?
> Alas! CONSUMPTION is her name."

This is the point to which I call your attention. It is a fact that the above nmmber die annnally with consumption alone, aside from other diseases, in America, and its mortality is fearfully on the increase; it is a fact, too, that not one case has ever been cured by giving drugs by the stomach! Will you, then, give your attention to the claims that a true system of treatment by inhalation has upon you to cure this insidious and fatal disease? whose terrible inflictions have rendered desolate so many thousands of happy homes; have laid low so many warm hearts and bright prospects; banished hope from our path and aim from life; a disease so all prevailing that its slightest symptoms is at once our first dread; such a disease, we say, forms so fearful a scourge that you would be inaccessible to the dictates of common humanity, did you not avail yourselves of every opportunity to direct attention to any circumstances, or remedial agent, offering the slightest probability of alleviating, in however minute a degree, its direful inflictions. It is highly consolatory to know that the influence of Medicated Inhalations at last bids fair to conquer its fatality. It should be remembered that every physician can give drugs by the stomach, but all are not equally alike successful; so all can give medicines by vapors and inhalation, but success will only be the reward of those who are meritorious, and whose powers of judgement and discrimination have been matured by years of hard study, close observation, and practical experience.

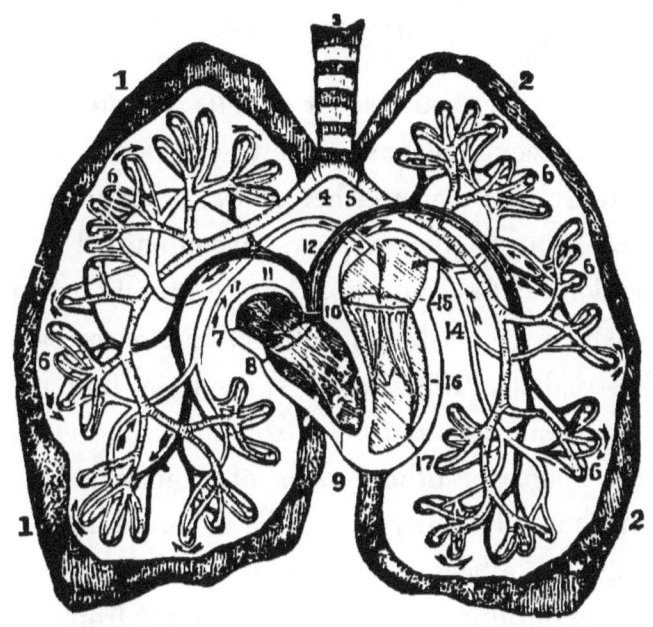

The Air-Passages of the Right and Left Lung.

CONSUMPTION:
AND ITS DIFFERENT VARIETIES.

CHAPTER I.

I shall notice only FEBRILE and LATENT. One of the most remarkable features of Febrile Consumption is the suddenness of the attack. The patient feels that he has taken a violent cold. He has a severe chill, followed by heat of the skin, quick pulse, and all the indications of a fever. These symptoms generally continue throughout the entire course of the disease, and are very liable to be mistaken for *billious* or *catarrhal fever.*

From the commencement the respiration is more hurried and quick than in either of the other forms of the disease. Cough soon appears, accompanied with expectoration, at first colorless, but gradually assuming a yellowish or greenish appearance, and occasionally we find it streaked with blood. We seldom find the matter expectorated mixed with softened tubercule, as in the last stages of other forms of Consumption. The patient generally sinks before the tubercular deposits in the lungs have become broken down.* Such is many times the continued severity of this fever from the commencement of the disease to its final termination, that the cough and other indications are liable to be regarded as only symptomatic, and consequently do not receive the early attention that their importance demands. Patients generally suffer more or less from pain in one or both sides, and not unfrequently an attack of diarrhoea supervenes, under the exhausting influences of which the strength rapidly fails, and the poor sufferer sinks down and dies in the space of a few weeks from the commencement of his illness.

Too often the attention of the medical man is diverted from the true character of the disease until it is far advanced. He now applies his stethescope to the chest, when he finds, alas! to his great astonishment, that his patient is in the last stages of consumption, and has but a few weeks at most to live. It is proper to remark that these difficulties in the way of forming a correct opinion are not always to be attributed to the carelessness or inexperience of the physician, but are many times owing in a great degree to the unwillingness of patients to believe that their lungs are diseased, or to submit to a thorough and careful stethescopic examination of their chest.

I have frequently seen patients, though filled with apprehension, go so far as to strive by every means in their power to disguise and miscolor their worst symptoms, in order that they might derive from their medical adviser a favorable opinion. Such instances are always to be deprecated, and the consumptive invalid should be warned, as he values life, never to pursue such a course. The most calamitous and fatal results may grow out of one single error committed in this way. Remember, my reader, if you have tubercles in your lungs, and they are not discovered until they are in their second stage, your case from being manageable and simple, becomes one of extreme doubt and peril.

We come now to notice in the last place one other form of Consumption, more insiduous in its advances than either of those already described. This is called "*Latent Consumption*," for the reason that tubercles exist in the lungs for a long time and even to a considerable extent, without giving rise to any of the usual symptoms indicating their presence, such as pain, cough, expectoration, or hemorrhage; nevertheless it is silently effecting its work of destruction, with as much rapidity and certainty as in other forms of Consumption, where the symptoms are more manifest.

As there is but little derangement of the general health, and no local symptoms that point to the lungs as the seat of the disease, the physician is seldom called to investigate the case until it has made considerable progress.

The physical signs and various symptoms relating to this form of disease are so obscure that the most careful scrutiny and closest observation on the part of the physician is required to detect its real character. So far from being always indicated by a cough, Louis, a French physician of great celebrity, has remarked that he has known the disease to exist in many instances from six months to two years without the presence of this most common and universally acknowledged symptom. When, however, the patient finds that he is declining in health, his countenance becomes pale or livid in appearance, and in addition to this he grows thinner and weaker day by day, and the food he takes affords him neither nourishment nor support. Though there be no cough, fever nor expectoration, he has good reason to be apprehensive in regard to his safety. The great probability is that tubercles already exist in his lungs, and, like the worm gnawing at the root of a tree, are silently working his destruction.

If, therefore, constitutional symptoms like the following: fever, emaciation, night sweats, diarrhœa, &c., do occur, the attention should be at once directed to the lungs as the probable seat of the mischief, since these symptoms cannot exist unless some local cause is present. And by instituting a proper inquiry and by making a careful examination of the chest, the scientific and experienced physician will seldom fail to detect the true state of the case. He will find dullness in the upper part of one or both lungs, generally immediately below the collar bone—a want of the natural resonance of the chest. The respiratory murmur, if not entirely wanting, will be feeble and indistinct. These symptoms when present point unmistakingly to the existence of tubercular deposits in the lungs.

In this connection there is still another point deserving of special attention. Tubercular disease of the lungs is very liable to be overlooked when complicated with *Dyspepsia*, the dyspeptic symptoms being more apparent than the tubercular. The patient having a pale and unhealthy appearance, loses his strength, and the food he takes, though sufficient in quantity, is not appropriated to the various wants of the system. These symptoms, in the absence of cough

4

and expectoration, he very naturally refers to a deranged state of the digestive organs. His family physician is called in, and prescribes the usual remedies for dyspepsia, but he finds no relief; his symptoms continue to grow worse; and while this course is persevered in, the tubercular disease is gradually extending, intrenching itself firmly in the system, and the patient learns when too late that he has been deceived—that he has only been attending to the symptoms of the disease, while the causes that have produced them have been suffered to go on undisturbed.

Sir James Clark, physician to the Queen of England, in alluding to mistakes of this character, observes— "We have known more than one example of extensive tubercular disease of the lungs discovered on a post-mortem examination, when during life the disease was looked for in the stomach or bowels."

I have been thus explicit in pointing out the different varieties of Consumption, because I painfully feel almost daily the pressing want of proper information on this subject. Scarcely a day passes that I am not consulted by invalids suffering from some of the various forms of pulmonary disease, many of whom have been told by their physicians at home that their disease was simply one of debility, or that their hacking cough and hemorrhage only proceeded from the throat, and that a change of air and of scenery would speedily restore them to health. Such are the heedless assertions daily made by physicians, either from ignorance or mistaken kindness ; and such the thoughtless advice given by many to friends whom they most dearly love.

In conclusion, I need scarcely say that a " neglected cold" and a " hacking cough," however trifling and unimportant they may seem, too often lead on by sure gradations to an early grave.

CHAPTER II.

HEMORRHAGE, OR BLEEDING OF THE LUNGS.

Spitting of blood is not uncommonly a very early symptom in phthisis. It frequently occurs before any of the well known symptoms of consumption are noticed, and when the individual by common observation would be regarded in a state of perfect health. It is sometimes very trifling in amount, a few specks or streaks are only to be seen occasionally in the matter expectorated. At other times, when the patient is least apprehensive of evil, a sudden and unexpected discharge of blood takes place from the lungs, even alarming in quantity.

Various opinions have been expressed with regard to the causes of hemorrhage; but from careful observation and inquiry into the history and symptoms of these cases, we have the most conclusive evidence in a very large proportion of cases that it is the result of tubercular deposits in the lungs.

The lamented and distinguished Dr. Swett very truly remarks, in his work on Diseases of the Chest, that whenever he is called to a patient who has bleeding at the lungs, he always marks him as a probable case of tuberculous disease. Persons under these circumstances are exceedingly liable to flatter themselves with the idea that the blood only comes from the throat; and I have ever known physicians themselves, from a mistaken sympathy or a desire to retain their patient, to encourage this fatal delusion, and thus allow the disease to pursue its fearful work without an effort to stay its progress. But let me say to those who have bled at the lungs, however small the quantity may have been, it speaks a terrible warning. We have strong reason already to suspect the existence of tubercles in the lungs. Beware then how you trifle with this important stage of the disease.

The reason why tubercular deposits cause bleeding from the lungs, is simply this: The pressure of the tubercles upon the small vessels in the lungs causes more or less obstruction of the blood in its passage through them, in consequence of which they become congested, and from over distention are ruptured, and a discharge of blood takes place.

Hemorrhage seldom proves fatal in its immediate effects. When this does occur, it is always in the latter stage of the disease, and then is the result of ulceration destroying some large vessel, causing a sudden gush of blood to flow out, and filling up the lungs in a few minutes, when death is the inevitable result.

I have already said that hemorrhage may be the first noticeable symptom of the disease. Again it may not occur until the disease is far advanced; and in a few instances it runs its entire course without a tinge of blood in the expectoration.

Andral, an eminent English pathologist, has given it as his opinion that hemorrhage occurs in about five cases out of six of those who die of consumption. Louis, a no less eminent French physician, has found it to take place in fifty-seven out of eighty-seven cases; Professor Walshe, of the London Consumptive Hospital, in eighty-one cases out of a hundred. It will be seen then that this is a very important symptom, and should in no case be disregarded. It is a very common occurrence, after an attack of bleeding at the lungs, to hear patients remark that they feel decidedly better, and indeed we not uncommonly find an improvement in all their symptoms. When the lungs have relieved themselves from the increased amount of blood which had accumulated in them, the chest, as a matter of course, feels lighter and more comfortable, while the operation of breathing is more naturally performed. This should not however be regarded as a removal of the difficulty, as at most it will be found to afford but temporary relief. The same causes that produced a hemorrhage in the first instances are still in operation, and will, if not arrested and removed by a careful and judicious system of treatment, assuredly lead on to a fatal issue. There is no time to be lost. Whatever is done must be done quickly. As you value health or prize life, begin now to resist the progress of this terrible disease. Do not wait, as is, alas! too often the case, until the grim tyrant has usurped his devastating reign over the system, when he may set at defiance every power to save.

The carelessness and reckless indifference with which some persons afflicted with incipient consumption have gone on from year to year, simply because they have not had all the symptoms which usually characterize this disease, has frequently been to us a source of most painful contemplation.

Those who know themselves to be exposed to the chances of pulmonary disease, cannot be too jealous in the watch they keep over the earliest perceptible signs of its approach. Let it not for a moment be forgotten that it is in the earlier stages that consumption is amenable to treatment, and curable as other forms of disease.

From this no one can fail to see that it is a matter of infinite importance that an early and correct diagnosis of the disease be made. A few careless thumps by an inexperienced and unskillful practitioner is not sufficient to detect the hiding place of the secret foe within. It is only from a most careful and thorough examination of the chest, taking into the account all the rational and physical signs of the disease, that we can hope to derive any correct or reliable opinion.

Sir James Clark, speaking of the many fatal blunders made by physicians in their examinations, says that he has known more than one example of tubercular disease of the lungs discovered on a post mortem examination, when during life the disease was looked for in the stomach, liver or bowels.

CHAPTER III.

ASTHMA, ITS CAUSES, SYMPTOMS, AND TREATMENT BY MEDICATED INHALATION.

This disease has from time immemorial been the subject of an almost endless controversy, but medical men pretty much all agree at the present time, that it is located in the mucous membrane of the bronchial tubes, and air cells of the lungs.

It manifests itself in paroxysms. These paroxysms generally come on at night, during sleep. The patient suddenly experiences such a sense of oppression and tightness across the chest as to occasion almost an actual state of suffocation. The lips become purple, the eyes protrude, and the countenance indicates the most intense anxiety and distress. The operation of breathing is performed with the utmost difficulty, and attended with a wheezing noise ; the patient springs up in bed, and calls for the windows and doors to be thrown wide open. In this condition he generally continues until toward morning, when the more urgent and distressing symptoms gradually abate ; the respiration becomes more natural and easy, a copious mucous expectoration takes place, and "tired nature's sweet restorer, balmy sleep," comes to his relief. Various causes have been assigned for these sudden and mysterious attacks.

The one which to my view seems most rational and conclusive is this: The air tubes or pipes which convey the air into the lungs are supplied with a muscular coat which gives them the power of contracting and expanding. It follows that when any irritating cause is applied to the nerves which go to supply this muscular coat, such as inhaling the fumes of arsenic, lead, or exposure to a raw, damp atmosphere, an instantaneous spasmodic contraction is produced, diminishing at once the size of the tubes in such a degree that it is impossible to receive through them a due supply of air to purify the blood.

It is wll known that most asthmatic subjects are peculiarly liable to gastric derangements, indigestion, flatulent colic, and various other morbid conditions of the stomach. This is easily understood, when we bear in mind that the *Neumogastric Nerve* presides over and forms a sustaining link of sympathy between the stomach and the lungs, so that any derangement of the former must produce a consequent derangement of the latter. Most asthmatic subjects bear a warm, dry air, better than a cold, humid atmosphere. Patients residing upon the seaboard are frequently much benefited by a removal into the interior or mountainous regions, and occasionally the very reverse obtains.

The benefits derived in either case seem to be owing particularly to a change of atmosphere. Asthma, in its early development, is rarely considered a disease of much danger, though it is by no means uncommon, where the disease has existed for a long time, for it to terminate in dangerous pulmonary congestions, disease of the heart, dropsical effusions of the chest, swelling of the ankles, and other symptoms characteristic of total exhaustion. The gradual inroads which it is sure to make upon the system during long years of suffering and anxiety are quite sufficient to embitter all the enjoyments of life, and make the poor sufferer look forward to the closing scene of his existence as the only hope of relief.

TREATMENT.

There is no disease more certainly under the control of medicine, and none which yields more readily to the action of remedies than that of Asthma. That medical men have failed in the use of the means hitherto employed for the cure of this disease, is to us not a matter of surprise, and if the same principles were to govern us in the administration of our remedies that have hitherto directed them, we too should have but little ground of hope. Their failure then is not so much to be attributed to the choice of the remedies, as to their mode of administration.

We contend that no remedy, or combination of remedies, however potent, whether *Allopathically or Homeopathetically administered through the medium of the stomach, has ever, nor can ever cure a single case of Asthma.* For the reason that they do not reach the seat of the disease, their principal force is spent upon the general system, and long before they find their way to the lungs, their power is lost.

It seems to us like the climax of folly to attempt to affect a disease in the lungs through the medium of the stomach, when by the simple and direct process of inhalation we can so readily gain access to the whole mucous surface and remotest air cells in the lungs, and bring all the active and medicinal properties of the remedy employed, at once upon the part diseased. Who that has observed the relief afforded to the suffering asthmatic by the burning and breathing the fumes of saltpetre, the smoking of stramonium, &c., can doubt the power and efficacy of inhaled remedies in the treatment of this disease, particularly when carefully selected and administered by the hand of science and experience.

These are the measures we depend upon in all Asthmatic and Pulmonary diseases; and we should just as soon think of *administering a suitable eye-wash into the stomach with a view to cure chronic inflammation and ulceration of the eyes, as to introduce remedies, however appropriate, into the same organ to cure a case of Asthma; since both are diseases of the same membrane, and depend alike on local causes.* I would not in these remarks convey the idea that all cases can and will be cured in which the treatment is used, but what I mean to say is this: that when complete disorganization does not already exist, and when the disease depends, as it does in a very large majority of cases, upon a morbid, irritable condition of the mucous membrane of the bronchial tubes, attended by spasms of their muscular coat, we regard it perfectly under the control of medicine administered by inhalation. And when the state of the disease has been such as to afford no prospect of a permanent cure, I have never known these remedies to fail in giving the greatest comfort and relief.

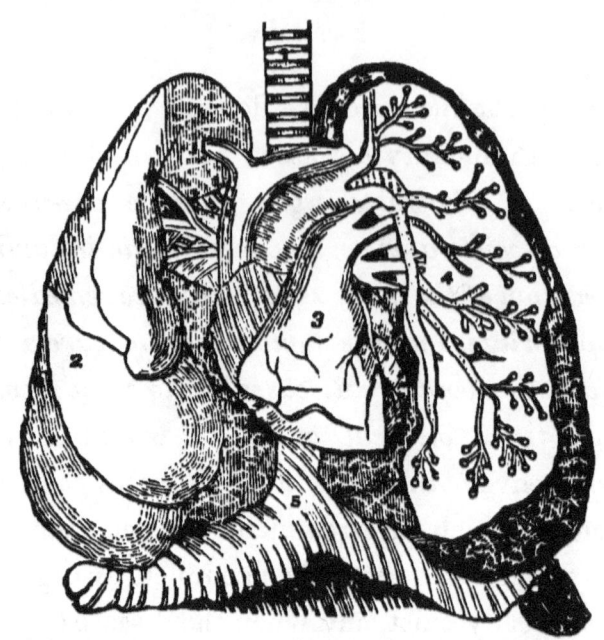

The Right Lung and Air-Passages of the Left Lung.

CHAPTER IV.

THE CAUSE, SYMPTOMS, PREVENTION, AND SPECIFIC TREATMENT OF CONSUMPTION.

There is no disease which has attracted so much attention as Consumption. From the earliest ages of which we have authentic records, the symptoms of this destructive malady have been remarked, and the causes producing it have been discussed. Nor is this to be wondered at; for the characteristics of the disease are so striking that they could not fail to arrest attention. The peculiar look, the gradual wasting of strength and flesh, the hopefulness of the patient, all tend to impress the mind of the most casual observer.

It is, however, a melancholy fact that, notwithstanding all the study bestowed upon it for so many ages, Consumption still sweeps off a greater portion of the human race than any other disease. It is confined neither to climate nor to race, and the inhabitants of the warmest as well as coldest regions, fall victims to its ravages.

When we find a disease thus universally prevalent, we naturally desire information as to its effects on the human race. Every one has known some friend or relation removed by this complaint, but there are few who will not be startled by the announcement that *one-fifth of the population of this country and Great Britain is swept off by its means.*

Scrofula, Consumption, and some other diseases of an equally fatal character, which arise from the same causes, and are of the same nature, may in a majority of cases, be prevented by a steady perseverance in a proper course of treatment. But, if diseases which destroy so large a portion of mankind, are so difficult of cure when once established, and are yet capable of prevention, how necessary it is that their nature, and the means of avoiding them, should be understood by the public at large.

It is now the general opinion of scientific men, that Consumption, in the first instance, depends upon a diseased condition of the blood; and that although most of the symptoms which characterize it manifest themselves in affections of the lungs, the difficulty of removing them hitherto has, in most cases, been connected with our inability to restore a healthy condition of the system at large, through a healthy action of the blood.

The blood, which is described in the Mosaic writings as The Life, performs most important offices in the animal economy. It affords the means whereby every part of the body is able to renovate itself, and at the same time, it sweeps away those portions of the system the continuance of which would prove fatal to existence.

Every one knows, from daily experience, that food is necessary for the support of life; but perhaps few understand the exact manner in which it sustains the body. In many instances, we are but little aware of the beauty of the arrangements that exist even in the most common things around us; and this is the case with respect to food, which affords the material for that wonderful process of REPAIR which is unceasingly going on in the animal frame.

Many may, perhaps, be startled by being told that every particle of their bodies is continually hastening to decay, and will probably be replaced more than once during their present lifetime. Life and death, growth and decay, are constantly going on in every tissue of which we are composed. The skin, which forms a covering to the body, in a healthy state, is constantly throwing off the dead particles from its surface; the muscles of the arm or leg lose a portion of their substance at every motion of their fibres; the brain, upon whose healthful action depends not only our own, but the happiness of others, suffers decay, in all probability, in every exercise of its power; and even the bones, hard and firm as they appear, are subject to the same law.

It is to supply new material for this continual *waste*, that food is taken into the body; and being digested, or converted into *chyme* by the *gastric juice* in the stomach, is received into and becomes a portion of the blood, and passing into each structure, affords the means of its renovation.

If the destruction of the different parts of the body is unceasing, so also is their renewal. Each particle, before disappearing, has its place supplied, and its functions performed, by its successor; and the blood, as it sweeps away the aged and worn-out portions, leaves in their room the materials for a new supply.

In order that the worn-out particles may be removed from the system, it is evident that they must first be reduced to a fluid or liquid form. This is effected by the oxygen contained in the blood, which by uniting with them, produces a *species of slow combustion.* Animal heat is caused by this process, and a number of substances are dissolved in the blood, which are afterwards expelled from the body by the lungs, kidneys and skin.

The tissues, or substance, of the body, for the most part, appear to be formed from minute particles, which are technically termed cells. By tracing the growth of these particles, or cells, we may comprehend the formation of the different structures of the body. The blood, when it first issued from its vessels, freighted with the elements necessary to supply nourishment to any part of the body, was of course in a fluid state. Part of it became solid, and the remainder was returned into the system by the veins. From the solid portion the cells arise, the first appearance of which is in the form of a small body, called the *nucleus*; around which a little bladder forms, filled with fluid, as in the skin, or as in the case of other structures, frequently with solid matter. In the structure of the skin, as the cell becomes older, other cells form beneath it and push it to the surface, by their growth. It becomes at the same time gradually flatter, until it appears as a thin scale, which, having accomplished its use, and its period of existence having expired, falls off. In the formation of what is called *cellular tissues*, of which many of the internal organs of the body are formed, the cells, instead of becoming flatter, are elongated, and their ends uniting, eventually form the fine fibres of which the structure consists.

By what power, it may be asked, does the blood pass through these various changes? This question can no more be answered than we can explain by what process the oak springs from the acorn, or seeds, which appear to us similar, should produce plants differing in properties and color.

Although we are unable to explain why, from the same blood, cells should arise which form tissues widely different in their nature and uses, we are, nevertheless, acquainted with certain conditions requisite for their development. One of these is, that there should be an adequate supply of blood; and another, that the blood must be of a proper constitution.

If the blood be so impoverished that the cells instead of being developed, stop short in the early stage of the process, it is perfectly evident that disease must be produced. This is the case in Scrofula and Consumption. And it is from this circumstance, apparently so simple, that such a large portion of the human race is annually swept off by death.

The structure of tubercle, in the early stage, is very simple. It seems to consist of a number of cells, which are small, stunted, and angular, and have often no nucleus within them; they are, in fact, cells whose development has been arrested; and they, consequently, show a want of power in the blood itself.

In almost every part of the body in which blood vessels exist, there is also an extensive net-work of other vessels, called *lymphatics*, or absorbents; the smaller uniting to form larger ones, until a few are produced which transmit the contents of the net-work of a whole limb. And again, these larger lymphatic trunks end by uniting in a single vessel called the thoracic duct, and which opens into a vein near the heart. The blood is supplied to the body by the heart, which forces it through a system of pipes attached to it, termed arteries. These pipes divide into very small vessels named capillaries, which again unite to form large tubes, called veins; and the veins, by being connected with the heart, return the fluid into that organ. As the blood is forced from the heart along the blood vessels, as soon as it reaches the small arteries, a portion of the liquid part of it oozes through their coats, and supplies the neighboring structures with nourishment (the remainder of the blood being returned to the heart by the veins), whilst the part not required for that purpose enters the small lymphatics, and is returned by them to the heart to be mixed again with the blood. There is thus a double circulation of the blood through the animal frame, the centre of both being the heart; in the one case the circle is formed by the blood vessels alone, in the other it is composed partly of the arteries and partly of the lymphatics.

In certain parts of their course, the larger lymphatic trunks are twisted upon themselves, so as to form what is termed a *lymphatic gland.* These bodies are placed in great numbers in the sides of the neck, in the membrane near the bowels, armpits, and other concealed situations. We might naturally suppose that in any disease of the fluid circulating in the *lymphatics*, the effects would be first observed where the twisting of the vessels afforded the greatest chance of obstruction; and such is found to be the case in the disease known as Scrofula, or King's Evil. In this disease, the tubercle, instead of being formed in the lungs, as in Consumption, is deposited in the lymphatic glands, and there produces the symptoms which characterize the complaint.

When tubercles affects the glands of the lymphatics leading from the bowels, a very formidable complaint is the result. Under such circumstances, there is usually long-continued diarrhœa; and as a great portion of the food ordinarily passes through the lymphatics of the intestines before entering the blood, in scrofula there is (as when tubercle is also deposited in the lungs) a rapid loss of strength.

When any part of the body is inflamed, the greater

portion of the swelling which attracts the eye of an observer arises from the liquid part of the blood which has oozed from the over-distended blood vessels; and in a healthy state of the system, certain changes take place, which prepare this liquid for being taken up into the blood as soon as the inflammation ceases. But in scrofulous constitutions, the blood has not sufficient vitality to undergo the necessary changes; and the formation of matter is the consequence. In those instances where the blood has not become so greatly impoverished, the scrofulous constitution displays itself by causing long standing inflammation of the eyelids, white specks upon the eye, inflammation of the nose or ear, or troublesome eruptions of the skin.

It has been stated that, in the destruction of the particles of the human frame, which is continually going on, they were reduced either into the form of gas or fluid, in order to be removed, or thrown off, from the body. The chief, if not the only gas thus formed, is carbonic acid.

All nature's works are fitted to perform the purposes for which they were intended; and in the human structure perhaps no organs display more beautiful design than the lungs; the perfect arrangement of their parts admirably adapting them for the performance of their important functions.

The lungs are two spongy bodies which, together

with the heart, fill up the whole of the hollow of the chest. They communicate with air by means of a long tube, named the trachea, or windpipe. This lies in front of the neck, covered only by the skin and fat, and reaches from below the tongue into the chest. In its upper part, it is closed by a valve called the epiglottis, which prevents food passing into the windpipe when in the act of swallowing. Below the epiglottis is the apparatus for speech, which consists of small cords, that narrow or enlarge the opening of the windpipe, at the will of the individual, through the agency of muscles attached to them. It is very common in Consumption, for small sores to form in this part of the windpipe; and a partial loss of voice is, in such cases, the result. Slight colds, by inflaming the part surrounding these cords, often produce the same effect.

The windpipe, after its entrance into the chest, divides into two tubes, which enter the substance of the lungs. Each tube immediately divides again into two, and is surrounded by the air-cells; and this method of division is continued until they attain a great degree of minuteness, and are distributed to every portion of the organ. These continuations of the windpipe are called bronchial tubes, which are composed of a firm substance, and are provided with muscles which can contract them; whilst they are lined internally with a membrane somewhat similar in structure to that which covers the inner surface of the mouth and throat.

Each bronchial tube terminates abruptly, by coming continuous with a membraneous passage, into which the air cells open on every side. It is named the inter-cellular passage, and is not lined by the membrane of the tube.

The greater part of the substance of the lungs consists of small cavities called air-cells, which give it its spongy appearance. Each of these cells is formed of the same membrane as the inter-cellular passages, and has no other lining. They are of different shapes, and communicate very freely with the neighboring passages, but not with each other. When inflammation occurs in this part of the structure of the lungs, it is called "pneumonia." In breathing, the air first enters the windpipe through the nose or mouth, passes through the bronchial tubes into the inter-cellular passages, and thence into the air-cells.

Having described the manner in which the air obtains entrance into the lungs, it will be proper to direct attention to the method by which the blood is brought into contact with it.

After the blood has traversed all parts of the body, and become loaded with carbonic acid gas and other impurities, it is returned to the heart.

By the contraction of this organ it is pumped into a

a large blood-vessel, which, dividing into two, carries the impure blood into each lung. The blood-vessels in the lungs, by continual divisions, attain a great degree of minuteness, and form a very close net work between the air-cells. By these smaller vessels being placed between two contiguous air-cells the blood in them is freely exposed to the air, by which a large quantity of oxygen is absorbed and the carbonic acid gas, produced by the slow combustion or union of the oxygen with the carbon of the decomposing particles is thrown off. After being thus purified by the expulsion of the carbonic acid gas, the blood is returned by the veins of the lungs into another of the cavities of the heart, whence it again issues to be used for the nourishment of the body.

The animal heat is kept up by this combustion of the decaying particles of the body, in union with the oxygen absorbed by the blood as it passes through the lungs, and carried along with it to every part of the system.

The carbonic acid, dissolved in the blood, replaces the atmospheric air which it before contained, and is of course, as deadly a poison when allowed to remain in it as it is when introduced from without. The use of the lungs is, therefore, to free the blood of this noxious gas, which, if not thus thrown off, necessarily produces death, the same as by strangulation.

It has been remarked that Consumption, as also many other complaints, originate in disease of the blood, and that, from the unhealthy condition of this fluid, a deposit of tuberculous matter takes place. The blood-vessels surrounding tubercular matter become gorged with blood, or in that state which is called inflammation. The tubercle, not being capable of forming part of the structure in which it is placed, excites the inflammatory action, on the same principle that any other dead substance — such as a thorn in the finger — brings on inflammation around it. The first effect of this condition upon the tubercle itself, is to fit it for being expelled from its position; and so far, therefore, a beneficial change is produced. Its substance becomes softer, and when examined under the microscope, its small cells are found broken up into granules. Whilst this is going on, the unhealthy inflammation is destroying the neighboring structures, so that when the tubercular matter is expectorated, by means of coughing, a hole or cavity is left in its place. From large quantities of the substances of the organs being thus got rid of, we often find the upper part of the lungs completely riddled with holes, or in other instances the cavities run together, and a perforation of enormous size is the result.

The important fact should be understood, that Consumption is a general as well as a local disease, and that other organs besides the lungs are liable to be affected during the progress of the malady. Consequently we find deposits of tubercle taking place in the glands of the bowels, in the membrane covering the intestines, in the brain and in other parts.

In more than half the cases of Consumption blood is expectorated, varying in amount from a few streaks to one or two pints. This blood is furnished by the vessels surrounding the deposit of tubercles. It is a symptom that should never be treated lightly, more especially if there be a predisposition to disease of the lungs.

The difficulty of breathing, which proceeds from the choking up of the air cells of the lungs with tubercle, is a very general symptom in Consumption. It is usually increased by the expectoration contained in the bronchial tubes, preventing the free passage of the air in and out of the air-cells. One of the most prominent and distressing symptoms of Consumption is cough; in the early stages of the disease the cough is short and without expectoration, and it often continues, without producing alarm, many months before any other symptom manifests itself. At this time it generally arises from the tubercle deposited in the air-cells irritating the nerves distributed to the lungs, but afterwards, when expectoration is present, it is, to a certain extent, useful, both in clearing the bronchial tubes and increasing the forcible inspiration that usually follows the act of coughing. Whenever a cough has continued more than a few weeks, especially if it has not been preceeded by discharge from the nose, or other symptoms of a common cold, attention should be directed to it; and, if the person so affected belong to a scrofulous or consumptive family, the greater watchfulness should be used.

Expectoration is usually not present in the commencement of the disease, the cough being dry and hacking. Afterwards, however, the cough is accompanied by a whitish, gluey matter, which chiefly occurs in the morning. As the disease advances it becomes thicker, often containing white particles, and in the last stages, it is usually in the form of thick yellow matter. In the earlier periods this matter is furnished by the bronchial tubes, and even at the last the greater portion is from this source. During the softening of the tubercles and when inflammation exists around them, the expectoration necessarily contains portions of the tubercle itself, and of the fluids thrown out from the vessels, but the greater part is always produced by the inflammation of the bronchial tubes.

One of the earliest symptoms of Consumption is the loss of flesh; and perhaps no case goes through all the various stages of the disease without it. It varies greatly in amount, in some instances being so gradual as to be scarcely perceptible, whilst in others it is so marked that it cannot fail to attract attention. Whenever a person predisposed to Consumption, becomes much thinner without evident cause—even if without cough or expectoration—his condition should not be neglected for a moment. *At this period prevention is certain, saving much suffering and perhaps death.*

My Inhalants in Tubercular Consumption is working wonders, in the ready mode of carrying its healing, stimulating and restorative action to every minute air-cell and branch of the air-tubes, relieving pain, calming irritation, arousing the malignant and ulcerated cavities to put on a healing process, and the absorbents stimulated to take out of the lungs the tubercular deposits.

It is a matter of great question to my mind if agents in the form of vapor alone will cure Pulmonary Tuberculosis from an hereditary cause, without the aid of nutrition and tonics, carried into the blood through the medium of the assimilative functions, to correct a scrofulous or bad state of the blood, the constitutional condition of which is the cause of the deposition of tubercles in the lungs. But the inhalation of these medicated vapors are a powerful auxiliary means even in this form of Consumption.

CHAPTER V.

CONSUMPTION AND ITS SYMPTOMS.

One of the most troublesome symptoms that occur in the progress of Consumption, and one that tends more than any other to weaken the sufferer, is diarrhœa. It often arises from weakness of the lining membrane of the bowels; but, if long continued, it is generally connected with deposits of tubercle and subsequent ulceration of the glands of the intestines. It is from this cause that this symptom is so difficult of removal and so often bids defiance to the best medical skill.

Hereditary Transmission, that is, the transmission from a parent to a child of a tendency to disease, is undoubtedly the most common predisposing cause both of Scrofula and Consumption. As these diseases arise from the same condition of the blood, it will be readily understood that they will both be produced by the same circumstances. This must be borne in mind, as from ignorance of it many persons deny that there is any tendency to consumption in their family. Scrofula,

Consumption, Gout, Rheumatism, and many other disorders, appear to be regularly transmitted from parents to children, and with them pain, misery, and often poverty.

A deficiency of proper food very often acts as an exciting cause to Scrofula or Consumption. When this deficiency of nutritious food is conjoined with a want of fresh air these diseases are exceedingly common. Unlike the deficiency of food, the want of air creates no craving or uneasiness in the frame, so that men forget its necessity, and bring on disease by over-crowding in dwelling houses, factories, churches, and places of public amusement. No part of the management of tuberculoses is of greater importance than that of Diet. Patients should live generously, indulging and cultivating an appetite for all the varied wholesome articles of food, with a full proportion of meat. A free use of sugar is also recommended by eminent medical authority. Diffusible stimuli, as wine, beer or Scotch ale, and even spirits, given in moderate quantities, tend to render the digestive process more active and complete. Patients affected with tuberculosis are often able to take spirits in large quantities without experiencing stimulating or intoxicating effects.

The hygienic influence of pure air cannot be overestimated by the patient. Frequent, or daily exercise, conjoined with agreeable mental occupation, exert a beneficial effect on the disease. As the advantages to be derived from pure air arise from its being taken into the chest of the individual, it is evident that any cause lessening the motion of the lungs must produce injurious effects. It is, perhaps, partially in this way that mental anxiety acts in bringing on disease, as every one is aware of the feeling of oppression accompanying this state of mind. The natural method of increasing the ordinary breathing is by exercise; for when the muscles of the body are put into rapid or violent motion the blood is forced more quickly through the lungs, and the air is more freely inspired for its purification.

In order clearly to understand the effects of the foregoing causes of Consumption, it will be necessary to inquire into the nature and healthy condition of the blood. When a drop of blood is placed beneath the microscope, a great number of small bodies termed blood globules, are observed floating in a thickish but transparent fluid. Two different kind of globules can be distinguished the most numerous being of a red color, and of a flattened shape like a piece of money, varying in diameter from one three-thousandeth to one four-thousandeth part of an inch. The other kind is much less numerous, there being in a state of health only one to fifty of the red globules; they being nearly round, and about one two-thousand-five-hundreth part of an inch in diameter.

The exact uses performed by these minute bodies have not been hitherto accurately known; but it is probable that their office is to carry air—oxygen—to the different parts of the body, and to prepare the fluid part of the blood for the nourishment of the various structures.

Sufficient is known to prove that *their presence is essential to the continuance of life;* and a redness of the face and lips, arising from a large quantity of the red blood-globules, is properly considered as a sign of robust health; whereas the pale condition of the skin, which may be observed where they are deficient, is always associated with bodily weakness.

As is the case with the solid parts of the body, there is a continual destruction and reproduction of the blood. The red globules after fulfilling their allotted period of existence gradually disappear by salution in the fluid in which they swim, whilst the white globules are changed into the red ones. These white globules, which are the immature red ones, are originally framed in the lymphatic vessels before described as receiving the contents of the blood-vessels, and their change into red globules appears to be chiefly produced by the action of the lungs.

It will, therefore, be readily understood that the fluid part of the blood depends for the continuance of its *proper constitution* upon complete *digestion* and *assimilation*; and, therefore, whatever impairs these indispensable requisites will be likely to derange the health and so give rise to the formation of tubercle.

There is nothing in which the public take a deeper interest than in the question, whether Consumption admits of a cure? The popular opinion is general, that when the lungs are once affected, the case of the patient is hopeless; and this opinion, we are pained to admit, receives too full a corroboration in the almost utter failure of the medical profession hitherto, *either to ascertain the cause of tuberculosis*, or to discover a *specific treatment* for it; but there is really no reason why nature should not repair an injury to the respiratory organs as she does to others less important for the carrying on of life.

It is admitted that ordinary inflammation of the lungs is *curable*; although the air-cells in this complaint are filled with matter, and cavities are not unfrequently produced. There is no reason for supposing that a similar happy result may not take place in Consumption; if the disease in the blood which gave rise to it, can be removed. However interesting it may be to prove that tubercle is curable, it is more important to the unprofessional public to know whether the complaint can be removed after it has reached to such an extent as to produce cough, wasting of flesh, and the other well known symptoms of *Decline*. There is no doubt in my mind that cure is possible, and that patients who present every mark of the complaint may be restored to health.

CHAPTER VI.

BRONCHITIS,—MINISTERS' SORE THROAT.

This very singular disease attacks a particular class of persons, those who are in the habit of speaking in public, and in crowded and ill-ventilated rooms. When it gets a fair hold of its victim it is a constant (although a very disagreeable) companion.

There has been much written upon this disease, and many methods of cure advised, but most of them without success. It affects the palate, tonsils, larynx, and bronchial tubes, and generally the digestive organs suffer more or less. Its progress at first is slow and insidious, creeping on the person step by step, until the whole phenomena of the malady are developed. Symptoms:—the patient complains of a constant tickling in the throat, as though something was lodged there, and he makes a great effort to dislodge it; but all his heming and coughing results in nothing but raising a small quantity of thick tenacious mucus. He feels better for a moment, and then the same disagreeable symptom returns, and the same hacking cough continues from week to week, hoarseness, a sensation of tightness across the chest, slight dyspnœa, acute pains darting through the upper portion of the lungs supervenes. On examining the throat you will find elongated palate, tumefied tonsils, and the whole mucous membrane congested and dry, the natural functions of the membrane to secrete healthy mucus destroyed. If the disease continues, the structure becomes thickened, mucous follicles enlarged, and the disease continues down the trachea into the bronchial tubes, and finally, if not arrested, tubercular deposits take place, and consumption terminates the patient's sufferings.

The stomach is primarily or secondarily affected, the tongue is covered with a white coat slightly tinged with yellow, and there is considerable nervous irritation, palpitation of the heart, disturbed sleep, and it is impossible to bring the mind to bear upon one subject for any length of time.

These and many other symptoms develop themselves from time to time as it progresses.

CHAPTER VII.

LARYNGITIS, CLERGYMAN'S SORE THROAT.

There is a modification of this form of Consumption which is a terror to the clergy and members of the bar; and as the author believes he has discovered a remedy which is almost a specific for this dreadful disease, he respectfully offers a few observations upon it. He means a disease of that part of the mucous membrane lining the larynx, giving rise to the clergyman's sore throat and consumption.

The disease is often extremely insidious at its commencement, and its progress is so tardy, that a great deal, and often irreparable mischief is done before any alarm is taken by the patient, or he applies for relief.

An uneasy sensation, and in some cases pain, is felt in the larynx, and extends over that organ, and at other times is restricted to a single spot; usually a tickling sensation exists which provokes caution, attended with a feeling in the throat as if there were something in the throat that ought to be removed, and feels raw. The pain is increased by coughing, speaking, inspiring cold air, or upon pressure being made upon the larynx. The voice becoming altered is frequently the first symptom that arrests the attention of the patient. It is at first weak, then becomes hoarse, and may suddenly or gradually be entirely lost, amounting to complete aphonia. The cough, in the first instance, is dry, but is afterwards accompanied with the expectoration of mucous mixed occasionally with pus or blood; often there are paroxyms or difficulty of breathing. The general health eventually begins to suffer. Emaciation, hectic, night-sweats, and often indications of tubercles, occur as the disease advances, and in the later stages, dropsical swelling, which increases until death.

EXCITING CAUSES.—Prolonged action of the vocal organs is generally the exciting causes of this disease; hence the disease is most common among actors, singers, lawyers, clergymen, &c. It is often wondered why the clergy are more liable to this disease than lawyers and professors are? The young clergyman, often of a feeble and nervous constitution, not only preaches twice or three times, or even more in a week, but is exposed to the night air and inclemency of the weather. He is compelled to do so, while the voice and constitution of the lawyer have generally full time for maturity before he need employ the one or expend the other, in the duties of his profession.

CHAPTER VIII.

BRONCHIAL CONSUMPTION.

This variety of consumption is the consequence, generally, of neglected cold. At first the symptoms resemble those of an ordinary cold or catarrh, the expectoration being tough, thick and opaque, but not yellow, containing small grayish lumps, which sink in water.— As the disease advances, the cough increases, and this tough mucous or phlegm becomes more and more mixed with a yellowish fluid, resembling pus or matter, and often slightly streaked with blood. In many instances the expectoration is of a whitish appearance, resembling cream, and sometimes a greenish-yellow color, which readily sinks in water. At first, the pulse becomes slightly accelerated and tense towards evening; and the heat of the surface of the body varies in the course of the day, being sometimes above and sometimes below the natural standard. Partial sweats occur in the head and breast at night. The thirst is generally considerably increased; the urine is highly colored, and deposits a copious reddish sediment; a sense of soreness in the chest, with an occasional transient stitch in the side, occurs in the majority of instances; but there is very rarely any fixed pain in the chest. The cough is unusually severe, particularly on rising out of bed in the morning, at which time the breathing is more or less wheezing, and attended with a feeling of tightness in the breast.

If the disease continues unchecked in its course the expectoration becomes purulent and extremely copious. Debility and emaciation increases rapidly, the difficulty of breathing and a sense of weight and tightness across the chest become more and more distressing. The pulse is now generally very frequent, being seldom under one hundred and twenty in a minute. In the early part of the day the face is usually pale, but a deep flush of one or both cheeks is commonly observed towards the evening. The tongue becomes clear and in many instances it assumes an alarming appearance, and is redder than in health. There are generally profuse and exhausting night-sweats at this advanced stage of the disease, and, unless relief is found, swelling of the ankles and diarrhœa supervene, and death closes the scene.

CHAPTER IX.

PLEURETIC CONSUMPTION.

This variety of Consumption depends on an effusion into the cavity of the chest, from inflammation of the pleura. While the effusion into the cavity of the chest is going on, the lung becomes more and more separated from the surface of the thorax, being gradually compressed by the accumulated fluid until it is reduced to a very small size, and more or less disorganized in its structure. While this is going on, ulceration sometimes takes place in some part of the pulmonary pleura and the corresponding substance of the lungs, and an opening is thus made into the bronchial tubes, through which the effused sero purulent fluid is discharged, by cough or expectoration. When this takes place, irritative fever, with night sweats, frequent cough, emaciation, and in short all the ordinary symptoms of Consumption supervene.

This form of consumption is generally the consequence of Pleurisy. It is characterized by a sense of oppression in the chest on lying down, difficult and hurried breathing in ascending stairs, or muscular exertion, short disturbed sleep, short tickling cough, aggravated on first lying down, spells of hurried and oppressed breathing after speaking, and generally more or less soreness of the external surface of the affected side of the chest. The patient is easiest when in a sitting posture; and if requested to take a deep breath while in the erect position, he will generally do it with little apparent difficulty; but when he lies flat down and draws a deep breath, he will complain of pain, tightness, soreness, load, or some kind of inconvenience in the chest. Death often occurs suddenly, and is almost invariably proceeded by considerable swelling of the legs and feet. In some instances, after the effused fluid is discharged through the lungs, the progress of the disease becomes arrested, and the patient recovers to a tolerable state of health. When this occurs the affected side of the chest contracts to a manifest degree, forming what Laenec describes under the name of contracted chest. Unless the progress of the disease is arrested, the difficulty of breathing becomes greater and greater, until at length the patient cannot lie down at all, and remains in this state until he dies.

For this form of Consumption, the effects of the inhalants are often surprising. Independent of its powerful expectorant effects, it possesses diaretic properties in an eminent degree, by healing and soothing the lungs and pleura; and with it I always give a Kidney Sanative which promotes the secretion of urine causing its copious flow, and the patient is rapidly cured.

CHAPTER X.

DYSPEPTIC CONSUMPTION.

When Bronchial Consumption is complicated with hepatic diseases, (an occurrence by no means uncommon,) it forms what is termed Dyspeptic Consumption. In this form of the disease we have in addition to the ordinary phenomena of bronchial disease, various symptoms indicative of hepatic disorders, such as tenderness and tension of the right side, irregularity of the bowels, unnatural stools, a sallow hue of the skin, and yellowness of the white of the eye, flatulency, indigestion, with variable appetite, increasing difficulty of breathing, and cough after eating hearty meals, furred and brown tongue, foul breath, nausea, and sometimes vomiting. In some instances of this form of the disease, no symptoms indicative of the pulmonic affection occur in the commencement of the malady, the only manifestations of disease being such as are usually present in liver complaints generally. A dull pain or tenderness in the right side, with increased uneasiness on lying on the left side, irregularity of the bowels, foul tongue and depression of the spirits, are in some cases the first symptoms complained of by the patient. The first warning of the disease in the bronchial membrane are slight. There is a slight cough, unattended with pain. By degrees the cough becomes more troublesome, and when it continues for some time a tough flem is expectorated. The breathing, too, is in some degree affected, and the sufferer complains of weight and tightnes across the chest. The bronchial affection now advances, until a copious purulent expectoration and the usual symptoms of hectic are fully established, which continues to increase till death ensues.

CHAPTER XI.

COUGHS AND COLDS.

Every case of consumption commences with cough, excited from the individual having taken cold.

The diseases of the air passages are of great interest to every intelligent being. The delicate organization of the lungs—their constant activity, and their being exposed to the contact of air of such different temperature, and which contains various irritating matters suspended in it, renders them especially liable to diseases, and those of a most serious character.

Let me direct your attention to the symptoms and different parts which are diseased when a person has a common cold.

The mouth, nose, throat, organs of voice, and lungs are lined by a continuous mucous membrane, which, in a state of health is constantly moist. The secretion of this moisture, to a certain amount, constitutes a necessary part of its healthy function; but when an individual gets a cold, a part of all this membrane becomes inflamed, the first effects of which is to alter its secretion.

It is at first dry—the secretion is suspended—it becomes swollen, and thicker than before—it is redder than natural and its sensibility is perceptibly altered. We can see a portion of this membrane, and by noticing the changes produced in it by inflammation, we infer those changes which are apt to take place in the parts we cannot see. Everybody has experienced, in their own person an inflammation of that part of the membrane lining the nose, constituting a cold in the head. At first the nostril is dry ; and though it is dry, we cannot breath through it—it is stuffed up by the membrane being swelled—the sense of smell is altered or lost ; the part is red, tender, and irritable ; the contact of air a little colder or less pure than common excites sneezing.

Sometimes, when the disease is severe, there is a slight chillness, and towards evening a little fever. After the dryness, the membrane secretes a thin, watery fluid, which by degrees becomes thicker ; the swelling of the membrane diminishes ; and as the inflammation subsides, it is less raw ; the secretions resumes its natural quality, and is reduced in quantity, and the membrane again is in its natural state. Such is the general course of a cold in the head.

When the inflammation goes down into the lungs, it is said to be a cold in the chest. It sometimes travels from one part of the membrane to another, beginning in the nose, and gradually creeping down into the windpipe and lungs. When a person has such a cold, there is a dry cough—more or less difficulty of breathing—sometimes a degree of pain or oppression across the chest, slight fever and thirst, and a thin white coat upon the tongue, which is not always the case.

These are the symptoms that usually occur in the milder forms of cold; none of which are troublesome but the cough. It is tight and dry; the membrane does not secrete, and nothing is expectorated. In this state, if a stimulating article is taken, how often does it drive the inflammation to the substance of the lungs; when tubercles rapidly form, and a person dies of the quick consumption.

I need scarcely say that a "neglected cold," and a "hacking cough," however trifling and unimportant they may seem, too often lead on by sure gradations to an early grave.

In no one point have mankind suffered more from the thraldom of physicians, than in adherence to the notion of poisoning the stomach with deadly drugs in Pulmonary Consumption, which, every intelligent person must know is a disease entirely local, situated in the chest, where drugs or medicines, when given into the stomach, could never reach; and still nearly the whole combined fraternity will degrade their reason and judgement so low as to pursue this course, so long as the poor patient will suffer himself to take the medicines;

and when about to die, he is greeted with the intelligence from them that consumption is incurable! But why prostitute reason and the noble science of medicine so low as to drug patients so long as they can swallow, and then show such inhumanity as to tell them that consumption is incurable?

Consumption is as curable as Dyspepsia, Liver Complaint, Diarrhœa and fever; only carry the medication and remedies directly to the parts affected, by breathing them, or inhaling them, in the shape of VAPORS, combining a nutritious diet, a due, rigid system of hygiene, of exercising in the open air, and the breathing of pure air at all times. Keep the patient buoyant with hope, and above all keep poisonous drugs and minerals out of the stomach. Under this system of treatment, consumption becomes as curable in our hands as any other disease; and we have the unbounded satisfaction of referring to hundreds of cases, snatched as it were from the jaws of death, after the combined powers of Allopathy had consigned them to the tomb. But we do this on rational and scientific principles, in accordance with the laws of health, and by aiding nature by carrying our medication where the disease is, and not by putting it into the stomach, where it is not.

CHAPTER XII.

A NEW AND ACCURATE METHOD FOR THE

DIAGNOSIS OF CONSUMPTION;

OR, HOW TO DETECT ITS SIGNS AND SYMPTOMS IN ITS VARIOUS STAGES.

We are well aware that the introduction of any thing new in medical science, will be subjected to the most severe scrutiny, especially if it conflicts with time honored notions, or individual interests; but we shall here give a treatise on the FAUCAL SYMPTOMS. In giving publicity to a discovery which we made more than sixteen years ago, and one which our experience has fully confirmed, in practice during this long period, we do not fear the severest scrutiny, coming from what source it may. Being convinced not only of its truth, and immense practical value to suffering humanity; but ultimate triumph over any and all other diagnostic signs heretofore discovered for detecting pulmonary phthisis; it will fortify us against the sarcasms of the ignorant and prejudiced that may censure us, being based upon facts its application is only required to demonstrate its utility. All we ask is a candid investigation, and we are willing to leave it with an intelligent public to pass their verdict, and abide its decision.

While this method will enable any one with the most limited knowledge to detect a disease upon the pulmonary organs, it will, nevertheless, require studious application, and not a little experience to describe their true condition in every respect.

There is no means heretofore known whereby pulmonary phthisis could be detected in its incipient stages, and this is the principle reason why it has proved so universally fatal. There is no necessary reason why this disease should be attended with fatal results, any more than a similar disease upon any other organ in the body—the medical profession have abundance of means at their command which enables them to detect phthisis in its last stages; but at this stage, were a similar disease located upon any other organ it would be equally incurable. Hence these means are of no practical value to the physicians, or their unfortunate patients. I do not wish to be understood as condemning, or entirely doing away with all other methods for diagnosing the disease in question, although they fail to admonish us of the existence of consumption in its incipient stages, they are nevertheless useful monitors assisting us in our diagnosis so far as they go. The old and established symptoms are so well known, especially to the profession, as to render it not only unnecessary, but superfluous to append them here, my object being rather to add to the facts already collected, than to supercede them. I confidently believe that my discovery is of more importance and practical value to mankind than any and all others of this age; and when once universally understood by physicians and people generally, pulmonary consumption will be as rarely seen as at any remote period in the world's history.

My discovery is based upon the altered appearance of the mucous membrane, of the fauces or throat. By observation it will be seen that this membrane undergoes various changes, in color and other appearances, just in proportion to the extent and severity of chronic irritation upon the lungs. It seems that Providence has wisely ordained these symptoms that we might be able, by observation and experience, to learn the actual condition of the pulmonary tissues. It is unnecessary for us to explain the "whys and wherefores" of these changes in this chapter—it is well known that certain appearances of the tongue indicate the condition of the stomach and other organs—at some remote period in the history of medicine, cognizance was taken of this fact, and the experience of after generations, confirmed and perfected these once new diagnostic signs. My notice was attracted to these faucal symptoms more than sixteen years ago from daily observations; from that time to the present, I have not had occasion to ever doubt its correctness. I am well aware that I have not by any means reduced them to perfection in every respect, but enough may be gleaned to enable any one to detect a diseased from a healthy lung. With regard to the various appearances this membrane may assume in the different stages of pulmonary phthisis, I am also aware that there is a field open for improvement, and to render it perfect in every respect may require years of practical observation and experience—yet by carefully observing the various changes pointed out in this chapter, will enable the physician to satisfy himself sufficiently for all practical purposes. The physician will be doubtless surprized at the frequency with which he will encounter these symptoms among the patients under his charge, many of which may be affected with other diseases, that will prove to be the immediate cause of their death. Many persons afflicted with pulmonary consumption often die with other acute diseases.

According to the late statistics, one out of every six that die—taking Europe and America together—are from diseased lungs alone; therefore, if he should find that one out of every six or eight of his patients had the symptoms herein described, he should not doubt the existence of pulmonary derangement in some form.

For convenience of description pulmonary consumption has been divided into three stages, between these no line of demarcation is accurately known, and, in truth, does not exist, and therefore the various changes which occur in phthisis is but one continuous chain of abnormal phenomena, modified only by the constitutional condition, habits, climate, and the medical treatment the invalid receives.

THE FIRST STAGE.

The first symptoms that indicate pulmonary phthisis, may be seen by examining the "Fauces," or back part of the throat, the mucous membrane covering those organs, presents a peculiar whitened appearance, occupying a space above and below the "uvula." The alteration at first is very slight, resembling a kind of fog, through which a slight reddish appearance may be observed. As the disease advances, the coating of this membrane becomes thicker, and presenting more of a snow white aspect, and at the same time extends over a greater surface of the fauces.

The above symptoms indicates simply a chronic irritation of the pulmonary organs, and is generally the only symptom that denotes any constitutional or local derangement.

These symptoms are present for weeks, or months, and

sometimes for years, before any others known to the medical profession manifest themselves.

At this stage of the complaint the recuperative powers of nature, will often, no doubt, overcome the disease in young and otherwise healthy subjects, as it does similar diseases upon other organs in the body; but to depend entirely upon unassisted nature, to say the least, would be extremely hazardous; like the viper in the wall, it might depart from your premises without leaving its deadly sting, but it would be much safer to destroy the reptile while in your power. In this stage of the disease where there is no constitusional predispotition to consumption, very little inhaling medicine would be required to restore the patient to a healthy condition; and when this is accomplished, the above symptoms will disappear, and the throat will present a natural and healthy appearance. But so long as the fauces present the appearance which we have described, just so long is the person in danger of Pulmonary Consumption and premature death.

From this thin and snowy white appearance, peculiar to the insipient stage of this complaint as the disease progresses, the coating of the fauces becomes gradually thicker, assumes a little darker appearance, and extends higher up towards the palate; and in some instances assumes rather of a redish color, in others tinged with yellow. In short, these symptoms are more plainly manifested in every respect, until the disease has reached what we may term the *Second Stage.*

The length of time occurring between the first and second stages, will depend wholly upon the rapidity with which the disease progresses, or runs its course when affecting different individuals. In some persons this disease proves fatal in a few weeks, in others it progresses so slow that months and years elapse before it terminates in death. In this stage of the complaint the fauces present, in addition to its peculiar color, a kind of furrel, and, if the disease is progressing rapidly, sometimes a darkish red or inflamed appearance. Usually at this stage of the disease, the back part of the tongue is more or less coated, with large "pappillia" about its roots, (yet the appetite in a majority of cases is unimpaired,) the fauces in most cases assume a slight cream-colored aspect, and as we before remarked, all the symptoms are more plainly indicated in every respect, until the third and last stage is fully developed. In most cases the disease is curable in the second stage if proper treatment is applied. Much will however depend upon the perseverance of the patient and his or her friends, and the treatment pursued by the physician. Unassisted nature never will overcome the disease when advanced to this state; and even the most judicious treatment will sometimes fail to restore the patient to health and strength. Many patients arrive at this stage of phthisis without any of those harrassing symptoms so familiar to almost every one who has witnessed the slow and insidious progress of this dreadful disease:—such as coughs, night sweats, pain in the sides, breast, shoulders, &c.; and even the stethoscope, in the most practical and skillful hands, may fail to reveal any disease upon the lungs. But whether the last mentioned symptoms are present or otherwise, it will require every possible effort of the physician and patient to prevent a fatal issue. Let no one whose throat presents the appearance described under the second stage, delay for a moment, but procure the best medical advice within their command; for without judicious advice, appropriate and persevering treatment, pulmonary consumption will put an end to your earthly existence.

THIRD AND LAST STAGE.

In this stage of the disease the fauces assume a peculiar yellowish or cream-colored appearance, and at the same time the coating on the membrane is somewhat thicker than in the second stage, and extending down the throat as far as the eye can see, and up too, and covering the palate; or in other words, the whole back part of the mouth and throat presents a slimy or glazed appearance of a light yellowish color. Whenever the above mentioned symptoms are seen upon the fauces, no matter how favorable the invalid's symptoms may be in every other respect, they surely indicate an incurable disease upon the pulmonary organs. We have known thousands of cases during the last eighteen years, where the above described symptoms were manifested, and have never been able to effect a radical cure in any case, neither have we witnessed one performed by any other physician, or with so much talked of improvement of the day. Yet we have cured hundreds who were afflicted with a racking cough, and expectorated large quantities of matter from the chest, and suffered more or less pain in the sides, breast, and shoulders, and night sweats, swollen ankles, &c.; but in all these cases the fauces presented almost a natural appearance in every respect. It is, however, proper to remark that in a majority of cases, where the fauces present the appearance described in the third stage of this complaint, most of the other symptoms so familiar to the profession are also manifested.

We have endeavored to point out the symptoms as they appear in the progress of pulmonary phthisis, in a manner that we might be correctly understood by all; and, although we may not have deliniated its appearance as it occurs in the different stages, so minutely and accurately as would be desirable, yet enough may be gleaned from the description here presented, together with personal observation, for all practical purposes;

and we will therefore conclude by saying that a white or coated appearance of the fauces, always indicates pulmonary derangement; and as this coating increases in thickness and color, the desease advances, or in other words the fauces is a kind of mirror by which we can accurately judge of the condition of the pulmonary tissues.

MODE OF EXAMINATION.

In order to examine a patient correctly, it should be done in the day-time; any other but a natural light is not to be depended upon. We never pretend to examine a patient by candle or gas light, the reflection of light is not so natural. It is true we might be able to distinguish a healthy from a diseased condition, especially in a well marked case; but to ascertain what condition the lungs were in would be a very doubtful experiment. We endeavor to seat the patient by the side of the window, so that the light will rest directly upon the fauces, and press down the tongue with an instrument, by which means we have a good view of those organs. As soon as a person becomes a little familiar with these faucel symptoms, he will be able to diagnose a case to his own satisfaction, almost instantly, without any of the ceremony alluded to in this chapter.

CHAPTER XIII.

AN INQUIRY CONCERNING THE NATURE OF DISEASE, AND A RATIONAL MODE OF CURE.

There are good grounds for believing that the great mass of human diseases (except the strictly surgical), in all their types and phases, are caused by morbid matter — matter alien to the healthy tissues of our organisms, which has either intruded itself through the skin, the air-passages, or the alimentary tract, or has been formed in the body itself by pathological changes, or physical decay. Reason would seem to afford support to this belief. Disease must have a material as well as an immaterial cause; that our brains, blood, or nerves are ever directly disturbed in their functions by spiritual causes, we have not the least proof. True, passions and mental emotions may cause disease, through agency of the nervous system, but in all such cases there is good reason to believe that some material change is effected in some of the elements of the body, which change is the final cause of the perverted function.

To illustrate. It is well known that mental influences will cause defect, excess or perversion of different secretions.

Excessive grief is not accompanied by tears; excessive fear stops the salivary secretion, and increases and perverts that of the bowels — jealousy and melancholy indulged, are supposed to vitiate the bile; Dr. Watson mentions a case of a young friend of his, who brought on himself "intense jaundice" from needless anxiety about an approaching examination in the College of Physicians, and adds *scores* of such cases are on record. The proof is very striking in the perversion of the mammary secretion — thus says Sir Astley Cooper: A fretful temper lessens the quantity of milk, renders it thin and serous, disturbing the child's bowels, producing intestinal fever and griping — this secretion may in this manner be so altered as to cause death; the following instances are of high authority. A carpenter fell into a quarrel with a soldier in his own house; the latter drew his sword upon him; the carpenter's wife first trembled from fear and terror, then sprang furiously at the soldier, wrested away the sword and broke it into pieces; after the quarrel was ended, and in a state of strong excitement, she took up her child from the cradle, where it lay playing in the most perfect health, never having had a moment's illness; she gave it the breast, — in a few minutes the infant left off nursing, became restless, panted, and sank dead upon its mother's breast. An English surgeon (Mr. Wardrop) mentions that having removed a small tumor from behind the ear of a mother, all went well until she fell into a violent passion and the child nursing soon after, died in convulsions. From these and similar illustrations, the inference seems justified that mental influences act as causes of disease, by inducing molecular changes in some of the elements of the body.

Further illustration and proof of the general materiality of the causes of disease may be found in the fact that several classes of disease are confessedly produced by morbid matter, somehow introduced into the body. A large number of types of fever are everywhere attributed to miasms. The cutaneous diseases known as the exanthemata, among which are measles, scarlet fever, and small-pox, are demonstrated by the common experience of mankind to depend upon an aura or virus, or substantive something communicable from person to person. In all epidemic and endemic diseases, the most rational induction has produced a general conviction that in a subtle or gross *material something*, lay the specific cause. Isolated forms of disease are confidently believed by good pathologists to fall into this category. Dr. Watson mentions a kind of asthma which he ascribes to some kind of emenation from certain of the grasses that are in flower about the time of hay-making. Scrofula and the matter of tubercle depend upon a malassimilation of the fibrinous elements of the blood. It is further an undoubted fact that a large number of morbid conditions of the body may arise from retention of the common excretions of the body in the blood from disorder of their separating glands. Drs. Watson and Williams speak of gout and rheumatism as dependent upon some morbid matter retained in the blood, and Dr. Prout seems to consider this as the lactic and lithic acids generated by imperfect assimilation. Bile and urea (secretions of the liver and kidneys,) are positive poisons, and when their elimination from the system is entirely suppressed they cause "typhoid symptoms," extreme depression and coma, which speedily end in death; and in these cases, and those of gradual suppression ending in death, the same excrementitious matters, which ought to have passed off by the liver and kidneys, can be detected in the solids and fluids of the body.

CHAPTER XIV.

GENERAL DEBILITY.

The term *general debility* is a convenient covering for a multitude of physiological transgressions.

At a season, when all animated creation save man is joyfully breathing from the frost-bound fetters of winter, it is a sad reflection upon *his good sense* to hear the almost universal complaint of general debility. Why should man be an exception in the united rejoicing? Endowed as he is with superior capacity for appreciating the natural changes, why do we hear murmurs instead of praises? Is it because the power Omnipotent has done less for him than for the rest of organic creation? No one believes this. Then let us look into the cause of this difficulty, and suggest a remedy therefor.

Man, unlike the brute, makes instinct a subordinate guide in the gratification of the animal propensities. He is continually committing depredations upon the laws of health, which render him as unhappy physically as violations of the moral law are destructive to his happiness morally. This is a case wherein the old maxim, that a little knowledge is a dangerous thing, holds emphatically true. Were man ignorant as the dumb beast, his appetites would not be guided by a perverted intellect; or, were he learned in the science of health and life, the voice of conscience would make him responsible for his transgressions. As the matter now stands, we find a vast majority of mankind attributing their physical sufferings to anything rather than their own ignorance and folly. Thus it will ever remain so long as parents and teachers deem it of more importance that their children become more familiar with the volcanoes and rivers of the earth, than with the vicera and life-streams within their own bodies. But to return to the causes which produce the general debility of the vernal season.

The long cold winters of our Nothern climate are anticipated by nearly all as fitting seasons for relaxation and social enjoyment. Few rely upon this season for pecuniary support. The farmer quietly pockets the pay for his previous labor, sends his children to school, and makes ready for the coming spring. The mechanic is content with smaller income, and has his long evenings for domestic intercourse and mental improvement. The merchant examines his stock in trade, balances his ledger, and hopes for a good " Spring business."

Now man is a busy creature, and it is easy to perceive why winter is chosen as the time for amusement. There is not much else to attract his attention. Social visits, balls, and parties are followed with even greater zeal than the plough, the plaine, or the sale of goods. No one questions the right to rich dinners, or late suppers; but during this "social season" it is downright vulgarity to talk of temperance, reasonable hours, and a healthful dress. To be candid, it is useless to enumerate the terrible violations of nature's law. When properly regulated, I do not by any means oppose the gratification of the social faculties; but as society now exists, a majority of people go on in this reckless manner, as though human life were a game of chance, and he who risks the most would be the greatest winner.

The result of this course of dissipation is not always immediately manifested. Trouble may not follow these excesses so long as the bracing or tonic effects of cold weather continues; but when the cool, oxygenated atmosphere of winter abates, and the "thawing out" of spring relaxes the system, there is nothing to sustain the body against the upheaving of morbific humors which have been assiduously deposited by the past few months' career.

There is loss of appetite, billiousness, universal weakness, giddiness, sinking sensations, palpitation; in a word, *general debility.*

These difficulties are not alone confined to the ranks of dissipation. All who *labor less* and *eat more* during the winter, sleep in small ill-ventilated rooms, upon feather beds, hazard that good health which, other things being equal, an opposite course would ensure.

In the treatment of these difficulties, it is customary to use, first. cathartics, and then tonics.

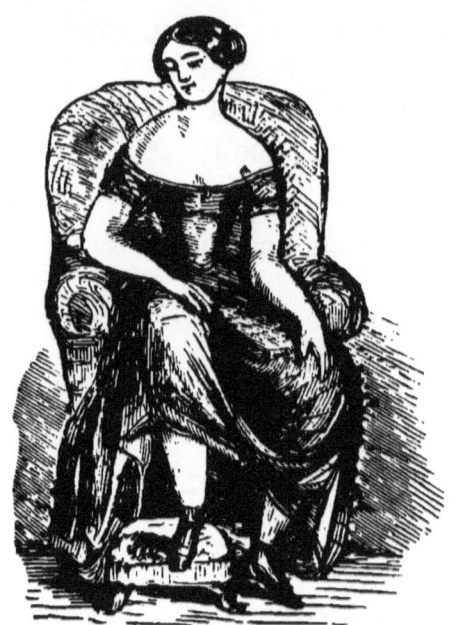

Healthy.

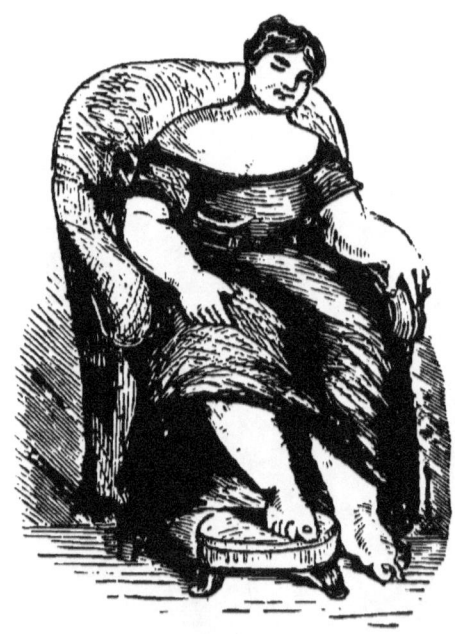

Dropsical.

CHAPTER XV.

THE SKIN AND ITS OFFICES.

In order to insure perfect health, great attention should be paid to the state of the skin. The skin is the external covering of the body, and is to man a natural clothing. There are yet some nations of the earth known to exist without wearing any artificial clothing whatever. I mention this as merely showing the amount of protection derived from the skin. That it is a covering or protection, we have only to notice those parts of our person that are exposed to the air, such as the hands and face, which are usually uncovered; these meet the air with perfect impunity. In addition to being a clothing, the skin is pierced with an innumerable number of very small holes, through which constantly pass a vast quantity of fluids from the body; either in apparent or invisible perspiration. Sometimes we will see great drops of perspiration standing on every part of the body; at other times it is not visible to the eye, yet it is always passing off in great quantities when in health. Were the clothing to be removed entirely from a man, and his body placed under a glass case, and the air pumped off, he would seem to be covered entirely with a cloud of vapor. This is the insensible perspiration. The same thing may be noticed on first entering a bath: in a moment or two after the person is under the water, upon looking over the surface of the body covered by the water, we will notice vast numbers of little air-bubbles, seeming to stick to the skin. The minute openings through the skin are called its pores, and through these pores vast quantities of fluids, and even solids pass off. It is perfectly indispensible to health, that the skin be kept in a healthy, vigorous condition, and that its pores be always entirely unobstructed. It is not desirable that the skin have too much clothing placed upon it; indeed, we should wear as little clothing as possible, consistently with comfort. This will depend upon each person's experience and early habits. It is well known to every observer, that those children who go barefooted through all the warm months of the year, and wear little more clothing than a linen or cotton shirt and trowsers would be upon boys, and continue this light clothing and bare feet for as many months as possible in each year, and during all the years of childhood, have much better constitutions, and enjoy far better health in after-life, than those who are more delicately brought up. The same thing applies to the continued preservation of health in adults. The more the surface of the body is exposed, and the lighter the clothing, if they can bear it, the more health they will have.

It is well known what excellent health the American Indians enjoy, and how impatient they are of clothing. For nearly or quite eight months of the year, in our cold climate, they wear very little clothing. For this reason, I think, cotton next to the skin is better than woollen. I will, however, leave this subject to every man's experience, fully believing that the less clothing we wear, consistently with comfort, is most conducive to health. I would particularly urge every man not to increase his clothing, unless forced to do so by actual suffering.

CHAPTER XVI.

DIET.

On no subject does medical philosophy fail more than on the subject of diet. This is so with the consumptive. I believe the best rule is, to allow them to eat whatever they please, without eating so much as to load the stomach or cause fever. Well cooked meats, fish, stale bread, vegetables, fruits, wine, beer, porter, &c., and in fact, every thing in moderation that gives strength and does not produce much fever; slight fever will soon go off, and does little hurt. Coffee I usually find to do harm, and also acids. Use a plenty of salt, not much pepper or spices. Salt provisions are not usually desirable. The food or drink usually, may be rather cold instead of very warm. Pastry and all varieties of confectionary, hashed, spiced, or sweet-meats, &c., should be used very sparingly. In all this the patient should be his own doctor, study his case carefully, and eat what he finds to agree with him, and not positively to disagree. Rigid rules of diet I have seldom found of much benefit.

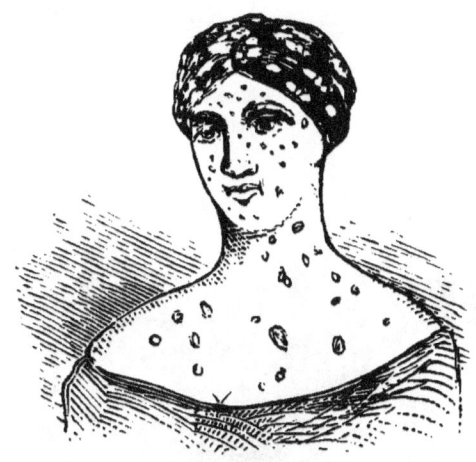
Scrofulous Humor.

CHAPTER XVII.

VARICOSE VEINS AND HUMORS.

Swelling of the Veins, or what are called Varicose Veins.—The same causes that produce swelling in the ancles, and feet, &c., will, in some ladies, though more rarely, produce swellings, greater or less, of the veins of the legs and feet. The veins, in some persons, in place of being the size of a knitting-needle, or a little larger, attain the size of a large goose-quill, and become hard, and run together in knots, feeling to the fingers like bunches of worms. These swellings are disagreeable, and at times dangerous. Instances have been known of these vessels bursting, and the persons bleeding to death.

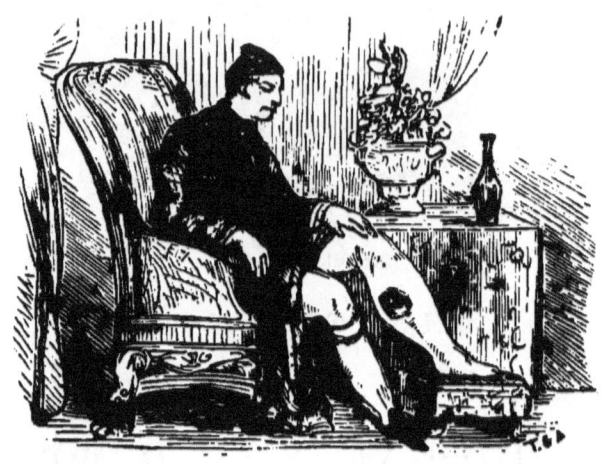

Bad Sores on the Legs, &c.—At times, very large, obstinate, running sores will occur on one or both ancles, or feet or legs. These sores arise from the same cause, in a great many cases,—which is a stoppage of the blood ascending through the abdomen. These sores can always be cured by suitable remedies.

CHAPTER XVIII.

HEMORRHOIDS, OR PILES.

The doctrine of nervous contractility explains many mysteries in the human economy. The fact that all functions are performed by the nervous energy, and that deprivation of the functions is the consequence of the feebleness of this energy, whether it results from waste, or is congenital, should be borne constantly in mind in contemplating our diseases. Our blood circulates to every tissue, and gives healthy nourishment, so long as the nervous energy in the coats of the blood-vessels is sufficient to contract the vessels, and send on the vital current. When this vital energy is lacking from birth, or from waste, we have feebleness and imperfection of function in different portions of the economy. Matters destined for the different tissues, or destined to be cast out of the system as effete, or hurtful, are left in organs where they do not belong—as the lungs, the liver, the spleen and kidneys—or they are left along the course of the circulation. So great is the waste of life, that there are few dissections of persons who are forty years of age, that do not reveal spicula of bone in the arteries. The bony matter is not carried as far as the bones, because the nervous power that circulates the blood is too feeble for the work. Our lives are so false, so filled with over exertion, and want of exertion, so unbalanced, so chained to the low and the gross, that life or vital energy is continually wasted, and imperfect performance of functions is the universal result. One is afflicted with dyspepsia, another has enlargement of the heart, or tubercles and ulcers in the lungs, or disease of the liver, or gravel, or piles; all these diseases come primarily from a weak and deficient nervous energy, which induces imperfect circulation. In piles, the coats of the blood-vessels, from the want of the nervous contractile power, sinks down into enlarged sacs. They become what is termed aneurismal. The blood of course moves slowly at first, like the water of a river where the bed widens, and after a time it becomes permanently lodged in these sacs, or aneurismal enlargements. A morbid deposition and growth is the consequence, and in extreme cases, no cure is to be had without excision of the morbid growth. After excision, the same causes will procure the same results.

The causes of piles are whatever exhausts the nervous energy. Some people say costiveness is a cause. Mechanically it has a bad effect, but piles and costiveness depend both on one cause: the want of nervous energy.

The use of drastic purgatives, of whatever kind, wastes the vitality of the nerves, and brings on costiveness and piles. The abuse of the sexual passion exhausts and diseases in like manner. The anxious, wearing life of our men of business, with their utter inattention to the laws which govern life and health, are fruitful causes of this weakness and disease. The cure must be in the use of means adapted to the condition of the patient. Where an operation is necessary, it must first be performed, but I believe it is often decided upon when wholly unnecessary.

The next thing is to give the patient a course of tonic treatment, if there is general weakness. If the patient is full of blood and life, and the weakness and disease are local, a *very spare*, plain, aperient diet, with morning and evening enemas of tepid water, and the use of the tepidsitz bath twice a day, and care not to perpetuate exhausting causes, will soon give relief.

CHAPTER XIX.

MANNER OF CURING COSTIVENESS.

As costiveness exerts such a pernicious influence upon the system and contributes so much to shorten life, it is most desirable to know how to prevent it. The best and most desirable mode of curing it, is by restoring the habit. Let the costive person, exactly at the same time every day, solicit an evacuation, and that most perseveringly for at least one hour, should he not succeed sooner, at the same time leaving off all medicine. So much is the system influenced by habit, aided by the will, that in nearly all cases obstinate perseverance in this course, and never omitting it afterwards, will entirely cure their sluggish state, and the bowels become as free as is desirable, and the calls of Nature become as regular and urgent as if they had never been interrupted. There are some persons, however, who seem, or pretend to believe, that they still require further assistance. These will find themselves greatly assisted by eating rather coarse food, such as coarse bread, rye and Indian bread, and bread made of wheat meal, or, we might call it, unbolted flour, sometimes called bran bread, and at other times Graham bread. Some persons derive great benefit from eating fruit. Almost all the summer fruits are found useful,—apples, &c.,—throughout the year. Others derive great benefit from the free use of vegetables, &c. All will be benefitted by avoiding the use of very tough meat, and very hard salted meat. I rarely recommend any other medicine to correct costiveness, than the use of a very small quantity of rhubarb. That which should be selected, if practicable, is the best Turkey rhubarb, either in the form of the root, or powder; the root is apt to be the purest. A few grains of this taken daily serves to improve digestion, strengthen the bowels, and remove costiveness. Rhubarb has the rare property over all other medicines with which I am acquainted, in a vast many cases, of never losing its effect. A great many medicines taken to open the bowels soon lose their effect, and require the dose to be very much increased; until, finally, they will not act in any dose, and leave the bowels much worse than when the patient commenced taking them. But this is not the case with rhubard, as a general thing.

In concluding this part of our subject, allow me to say to you, that to have the bowels in perfect order, and acting freely and kindly every day, is most desirable, and may be said to be indispensable to health and long life, and with this the happiness, the delights, and the pleasures of existence. A free, healthy state of the bowels is truly a pearl of great price, and a condition of inestimable value to the possessor. It is true, that some persons of costive habits live to old age, whilst thousands and tens of thousands are destroyed by it. The fact only proves under what disadvantages the system will labor on, and continue its functions. Let me repeat that HABIT, HABIT, is the great cure-all. Assist this, if necessary by regulating the diet, and, as a last resort, use a little rhubarb,—but assist all by habit.

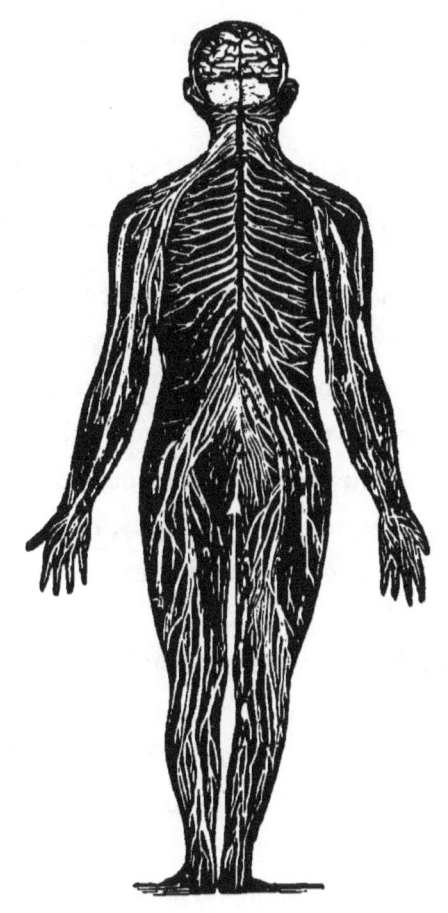

The Nervous System.—View of the Brain and Nerves

CHAPTER XX.

CHRONIC DISEASES, ESPECIALLY THE NERVOUS DISEASES OF WOMEN.

Who does not know that there are diseases of which almost every one in life is suffering, more or less; diseases which follow many to their graves, diseases which, because of their universality, attract little or no attention?

Who is not surprised at witnessing the daily increase of hospitals, medical colleges, men, and books, and at the same time the frightful increase of human maladies?

Whose heart is not filled with pity to see mankind suffering under such a burden of distempers, when he reflects that man came from the hands of his Creator as perfect and as healthful as the beast of the forest and the bird of the air?

Who has not often heard the assertion, that all these evils are inseparably connected with the progress of civilization, while their true cause is in the violation of nature's laws? And who does not conclude that the judgment of civilized mankind must be erroneous, when digression from the path of nature is entitled "The progress of civilization," while at the same time medicines are resorted to, in order to correct the consequences of their imprudence, and neutralize their follies?

True civilization must preserve the health of man, and make him happier; it must in every respect elevate him above the brute, and its progress must not bring him incessantly nearer to his dissolution, as has been the case with all nations which history has seen emerged from a state of barbarism, and passing through one of sickly refinement, into one of premature decay.

The chronic diseases, and especially those so called nervous diseases of women, are so various and so life-embittering, as to have always engaged a large share of the attention of medical practitioners; and very properly so, since we may safely say, that one half of all human misery would be removed, could these be annihilated, or even overcome.

It is melancholy to contemplate those terrible hysterical disorders, those hydra-headed monsters, which transform the dwellings of so many happy families into the abodes of misery; those giants, which have for centuries withstood all the orthodoxy of the schools, and not only withstood, but grown more luxurious daily; and which, when overcome in one form, assume ten new ones for the emergency. They are beyond description, and being so variously disguised are seldom recognized, and thus exert an influence of incredible power.

If we knew that hysterics manifest themselves, according to their violence and circumstances, in the form of excessive tenderness, false sensibility, fear, pride, jealousy, disposition to slander, discontentedness, quick temper, revenge, intolerance, hypocrisy, untruth, inconsistency, weakness of mind, delirium, etc.; that they are accompanied by heat, congestion of blood in the head, cramps convulsions, cold, chills over the body, sleeplessness at night and drowsiness by day, want of appetite, faintness, exhaustion, palpitation of the heart, and an infinite chain of morbid symptoms—if we consider these facts, we shall have the key to those ridiculous scenes, peevishness, and discord which are so frequent in married life, and which so often sap the foundations of domestic happiness; and we shall ascertain that not the hysterical woman, but the one who is not so, forms the exception to the rule.

The wide-spread existence of these affections, which are to be met with, more or less, in every family, makes a woman (physically speaking) always a mystery, and produces those bitter disappointments which are so often the subject of regret, and lead us to imagine that God has constituted woman incapable of the office which nature has assigned her, as no collateral agents can avail in correcting their deleterious influences, no scholar can explain their existence, and none of the countless treatises, which centuries have produced, can afford relief.

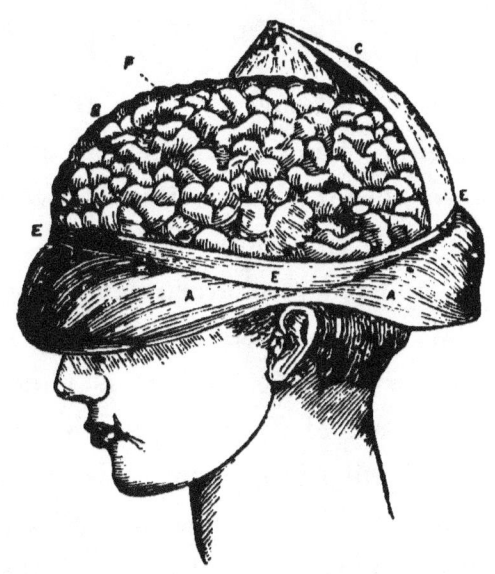

The Brain, as it lies in the skull, exposed to view, the dura matter, which envelops the brain and lines the skull, being raised by a hook.

CHAPTER XXI.

EPILEPSY, OR FITS.

This is one of the most horrible diseases that afflict mankind, and it is not surprising that, in ignorant ages, in Rome, in Egypt, and elsewhere, epileptics were considered as having excited the ire of the Divinity, or as possessing supernatural powers, on account of which they were worshiped. This was due to the violence and extraordinary force developed by the muscles in epileptic convulsions; the screaming, the changes in color, and the contortions of the face, the biting of the tongue, followed by a comatose state and afterward by a degree of mental alienation There are so many varieties of epilepsy that it is impossible to give a definition of the disease that will apply to them all. However, in most cases, epilepsy is characterized by convulsions and loss of consciousness, occuring at long or short intervals, during which the patient is almost in good health. The absence of fever in epileptics serves to distinguish their affection from meningitis and other inflamations accompanied by convulsions. The loss of consciousness also distinguishes epilepsy from hysteria. As in most nervous diseases, a hereditary tendency is among the most frequent predisposing causes of epilepsy. Leuret and Delasiauve endeavour to show that it is very rarely inherited; but the testimony of many others leaves no doubt about the frequency of this predisposing cause. Epilepsy often appears in the offspring of persons who have had various other nervous complaints. Bouchet and Cazauvichl say that out of 130 epileptics 30 were descendants of persons who had been either epileptic, insane, paralytic, apoplectic, or hysteric. As regards the predisposing influence of sex, there is no doubt that women are much more frequently attacked by epilepsy than men. As regards the influence of age, we find by a comparison of the statistics given by several English and French authorities, that the most frequent periods of life at which epilepsy begins are early infancy and the age of puberty. Epilepsy often appears also in very old age; Delasiauve remarked that out of 285 epileptics the disease began in 10 when they were from 60 to 80 years old. In fact, there is no age that escapes. As regards climate, nothing very positive has been established, but it seems probable that the disease is more frequent in hot and in very cold than in temperate climates. Although we have no scientific data to rely upon, we think that the extreme variations of the climate of the United States are among the causes of the greater frequency of epilepsy in this country than in England, France and Germany. Herpin, with others, states that epilepsy is more common in persons of low stature; but even if this be true, Herpin is wrong in considering the shortness of stature a predisposing cause of the disease, as in many of the cases on which he grounds his view it is partly the influence of epilepsy, already existing in childhood, or in adolescence, that has prevented the developement of the body. Various malformations of the body, and especially of the cranium, are certainly among the most frequent predisposing causes. Weak constitutions, as proved by Esquirol, and lately by Dr. C. B. Radcliffe, are favorable to the production of epilepsy. Among other predisposing causes are dentition, the first appearance and the cessation of menstruation, onanism, and the abuse of alcoholic drinks. Almost all kinds of diseases may produce epilepsy, but among the principal we must place those affections in which the blood becomes altered or diminished in its amount, and organic affections of the membranes of the cerebro-spinal axis and of certain parts of this nervous centre. Another very powerful cause, the influence of which has been demonstrated by Marshall Hall and recently by Kussmaul and Jenner, and by Brown-Séquard, is excessive loss of blood. Pregnancy, parturition, and menstruation, frequently cause epilepsy. A tumor on a nerve, or any cause of irritation on the trunk or the terminal part of any sensitive nerve, and especially in the skin or a mucous membrane, very often produces it. A wound, a burn, worms in the bowels or elsewhere, stone in the bladder or in other places, a foreign body in the ear, &c., are known to have caused epilepsy. It is quite certain that great mental excitement or emotion has originated epilepsy in many cases, but it seems probable that the disease was not produced by those causes, but has only been brought to manifest itself by this kind of excitement. When a complete fit is about to take place, it is usually preceeded by some sensation or some change in the mind of the patient. If a sensation precedes the fit, it comes more frequently from some part of the skin, and especially from that of the fingers and toes. This sensation is well known under the name of *aura epileptica*. There is as much variety as regards the kind and the intensity of the sensation as there is in respect to its point of starting. Most frequently, however, the aura is a sensation of cold, of burning, or that kind of sensation produced by a draft of cold air on a limited part of the body. Sometimes the aura starts from the eye or the ear, and then a flash of light or some other sensation comes from the retina, or peculiar sounds are heard. Some epileptics become gay, others mournful, when they are about to have a fit; in others the attack is announced by some change in the digestive functions. Whether preceded or not by an aura or by any change in the functions of the various organs, a complete attack usually begins with an extreme paleness of the face, and at the same time, or nearly so, there are contractions of several muscles of the face, the eye, and the neck. Observers do not agree as regards the first manifestation of a fit, probably because the seizure does not always begin with the same phenomenon. Not only have we known the first symptom not to be the same in different epileptics, but in the same one we have seen differences in this respect in three different attacks.

Some epileptics certainly are exceptions to the rule advanced by Dr. C. J. B. Williams, which is that the first manifestation of an attack is a palpitation of the heart. Many physicians think the scream is the first symptom. It often is, but paleness of the face usually precedes it. Some epileptics do not scream. As soon as these symptoms have appeared, a rigid tetanic or at least tonic spasm takes place in the limbs, and the patient falls. Respiration is suspended, and the face becomes quite injected with black blood, and assumes a hideous aspect both from the spasms of its muscles and the blackish or bluish hue. Sometimes a momentary relaxation is then observed in the limbs; but almost at once chronic convulsions occur everywhere in the trunk, the limbs, the face, and often in the various internal organs of the bladder, the bowels, and even in the uterus. The mouth then ejects a frothy saliva, often reddened with blood from the bitten tongue. The respiratory muscles, after the first spasms which produce the scream and suffocation, causing a gurgling or hissing sound, become relaxed, and then those employed in inspiration contract, and almost as soon as air has reached the lungs the convulsions cease or notably diminish. Ordinarily the fit is over in a few minutes; but it is not unfrequently the case that after a general relaxation another seizure comes on, and sometimes many occur with very short intermissions. During the whole time the fit lasts the patient is deprived of consciousness, and when he recovers he remembers nothing that has taken place in the mean time. In some cases the seizure is followed by a prolonged coma, ending sometimes in death. When the patient recovers from a fit, even if it has not been a very severe one, he usually feels extremely fatigued and suffers from headache. Fortunately, however, he soon falls asleep, and ordinarily is almost as well as usual when he wakes up, except that the headache and the fatigue still exists, though much diminished. When many fits have taken place, even at somewhat long intervals, such as several weeks, mental derangement often supervenes, and in this way epilepsy leads to insanity. In some cases the fits recur at regular periods; in others they return with every return of the circumstances which seem to have caused the first, such as menstruation, pregnancy, the influence of certain seasons, &c. There is seldom great regularity in the length of the intervals between the fits, and they come every day, every week, every month, &c., at irregular hours. Many patients have very different intervals between their successive fits. Some have many fits a day, others one every six months, or every year. Delasiauve mentions a case in which the number of fits was 2,500 in a month. But the greater the number of fits the less violent they generally are.

We have already said that the varieties of epilepsies are numerous; and among them the two principal especially require to be noticed. In a complete fit of epilepsy there are two distinct features : 1, the loss of consciousness; 2, the muscular convulsions. Each of these may exist alone. In the case of a seizure consisting only of a loss of consciousness without convulsions, we have the so-called epileptic vertigo, which is a form of epilepsy that frequently exists alone, and also co-exists often with the form of the disease in which the attack is complete. In this last case the patient sometimes has a complete seizure, sometimes only a more or less prolonged attack of vertigo. Whether vertigo exists alone or co-exists with complete attacks, it is a very dangerous affection, not for the life of the patient, but because fits of simple vertigo lead more frequently to insanity than complete fits of epilepsy. The cases of epileptiform convulsions without loss of consciousness are not so frequent as the cases of simple vertigo. They are particularly produced by injuries to the nerves or to the spinal cord.

The nature of epilepsy, the material and dynamical conditions of the parts which are affected in the animal organism, have been greatly illustrated by the researches of modern physiologists and practitioners. Dr. Marshall Hall thought the seat of epilepsy to be chiefly in the medula oblongita, and that its nature consisted in an increased reflex power, at least in the beginning of the disease, and also that the convulsions were the results of the asphyxia caused by the closure of the larynx (*laryngismus*). This theory is in opposition to several facts. In the first place, although laryngismus almost always exists, there is one kind of convulsions (the tonic) which precedes the asphyxia. Beside, there are more powerful causes of asphyxia in the condition of circulation in the brain and the spasm of the muscles of the chest. Then, as regards the increased reflex power, Dr. Hall acknowledges that this power is diminished in persons who have been epileptic for some time. We cannot admit, therefore, that the disease consists in the increase of this power. Another theory has been recently proposed by Brown-Séquard. Guided by experiments on animals, in which he produces epilepsy, he has found that the reflex power is composed of two distinct powers, one of which he calls the reflex force and the other the reflex excitability. He has found that the reflex force may be very much diminished while the reflex excitability is very much increased. This last power is the power of impressibility of the cerebro-spinal axis; in epileptics this impressibillity is very much augmented. The slightest excitations may produce reflex actions in them. In the beginning of epilepsy, usually the other reflex power, which is the force manifested in the reflex actions of the cerebro-spinal axis, is increased; but after a time this force diminishes, and in most cases it becomes less, and even much less, than in healthy people. Now the nature of epilepsy seems to consist in an increase of the impressibility, or, in other words, of the reflex excitability of certain parts of the cerebro-spinal axis. In most cases of epilepsy these parts are the medulla oblongata and the neighboring parts of the encephalon and of the spinal cord. But the seat is not constant, and may be sometimes limited to the oblong medulla or extended to other parts of the cerebro-spinal axis.

Dr. Brown-Séquard has tried to explain this mysterious phenomenon of loss of consciousness. It seemed very strange that at the same time that certain parts of the encephalon were acting with great energy, another part should be completely deprived of action. This, according to the above named writer, is very simple. The blood vessels of that part of the brain which is the seat of consciousness and of the mental faculties, receive nerves from the medulla oblongata and the spinal cord; these blood vessels, when they are excited, contract and expel the blood they normally contain, and it is known that all the functions of that part of the brain cease when they do not receive blood. Now, when the excitation that exists in the beginning of a fit acts upon the medulla oblongata and its neighborhood, it produces at the same time the contraction of the blood vessels and of that part of the brain which we have mentioned, and a convulsive contraction of the muscles of the face, the eye, the neck, the larynx, &c., all parts receiving nerves from the same source as these blood vessels. In this way the loss of consciousness is explained.

The first thing to be done for an epileptic is to find out the cause of the disease, and to try to get rid of that cause if it still exists. Very often epilepsy depends upon some external cause of irritation which may easily be removed; it is of the greatest importance to discover if there is anywhere such an irritation, and as the patient may not be aware of its existence, it is necessary to look for it everywhere. Of the various modes of treatment, the most powerful are those means of exciting the skin which most readily produce a change in the nutrition of the encephalon and spinal cord. All physicians know what these means are. One of the most efficacious remedies is belladonna. Physicians should not despair of curing their patients, and should not change a mode of treatment until they have given it a fair trial; and patients and their families should remember that the rules of hygiene must be followed by epileptics much more closely than by those afflicted with almost any other disease.

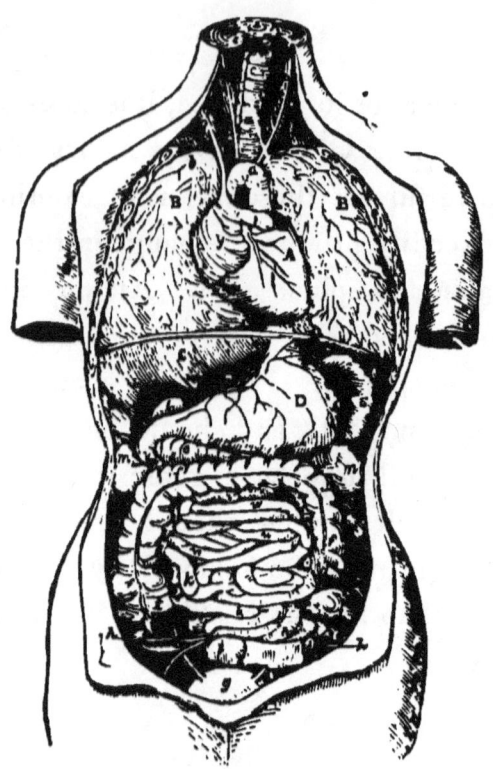

THE INTERNAL ORGANS.

CHAPTER XXII.

THE STOMACH.

I will remark that, the stomach has a good deal the form of a hunter's horn, its larger portion being towards the left side, at the upper part of the abdomen, and separated from the heart and lungs by the midriff, or diaphragm, which is a fleshy curtain that divides the abdomen from the chest. (See *D* in plate of Internal Organs.) The inlet to the stomach is on the top, at its left side; the outlet is at its right end; much the larger portion of the stomach hangs below its outlet. This arrangement prevents the food and liquids from passing out of the stomach, by their simple weight alone. The stomach will hold from one pint to two quarts. Its walls are very thin, generally, and are capable of being very considerably stretched. This is one of the causes of its difference in size. Those who eat and drink a great deal at a time, are apt to have much larger stomachs than moderate eaters and drinkers. The food remains in a healthy stomach from half an hour to four hours. As soon as food is swallowed, there commences a process by which a considerable portion of it is eventually converted into blood. This, considered in all its steps, is one of the most mysterious processes known to us. How portions of a potatoe, for instance, can be so modified and changed as to become flesh, is very difficult of explanation. We know it takes place, but exactly how, is difficult to determine.

It is the purpose of the lungs to give us the power of action, whilst it is the duty of the stomach to make such changes in the food, that this shall form the substance and growth of the body, and serve to repair all the waste of the body. It is of vast assistance to our stomachs, that the food is well chewed or ground up before it is swallowed, so that when it comes into the stomach, it shall be in a state of fine, minute divison. When the stomach is unhealthy, food may remain in it a great length of time. Thus in weak stomachs the food may remain a long time without being much changed; or it may ferment and form a strong acid, at the same time generating air more or less foul, at times producing an exceedingly unpleasant breath. These unnatural changes and decay of the food in the stomach, attend the disease called *dyspepsia*. This is occasioned by various causes, but chiefly in grown-up persons it arises from badly masticating the food, from debility of the stomach itself, but above everything, and more than all other causes combined, it arises from eating more than the waste of the system requires. For we must always bear in mind, that after the human frame is fully formed, all the object and purpose of food is to repair its waste, or the loss of its substance which is daily taking place. Now, the system, when not under the influence of disease, experiences the greatest waste and loss of substance by hard and long-continued labor, such as is experienced by all the out-door laboring population, and by many in-door laborers. Hard and long-continued out-door labor, unless too excessive, greatly invigorates the system, improves the appetite, and strengthens the stomach, at the same time producing great waste of the substance of the body; the stomach, now greatly invigorated, is called upon to furnish the supplies, to repair all this waste; it is under these circumstances that the stomach is able to do its best performances; it seizes upon any, even the plainest and coarsest, food and rapidly converts it into materials for the healthiest blood, so that the waste of the person of the laboring man is promptly repaired. So active is his stomach, that he is obliged to eat coarse and hearty food, that it may not pass off too rapidly. Now, the idle, the effeminate, and all those that pursue sedentary occupations, experience but a small share of the waste of the body that is suffered by the laboring man. Hence it is, that they are called upon to eat vastly less food and much lighter in its quality, and easier of digestion, than the laboring man.

The great secret of preventing dyspepsia is never to eat any more than the waste of the body requires. How much or how little this is, can only be determined by the experience of each individual. There is no laying down any positive rules on this subject. Each individual will learn, that if he eats, even for a short period, more food than the waste of the system requires, or its growth demands, the stomach may at first digest this surplus food, but in a short time, as if possessed of an intuitive perception that these extra surpluses are not wanted, it will refuse to prepare them; refusing, of course, to digest this surplus quantity of food.

Progress of the Food after leaving the Stomach.— The food, after remaining in a healthy stomach from half an hour to four hours, passes out of the right opening of the stomach. The process of digestion having reduced the food to a homogeneous consistence, very much like cream in its substance, after leaving the stomach and going a short distance, it unites with bile. A portion of stimulants and liquids go from the stomach into the blood.

The bile is as bitter as soap, the object of which is to produce still further change in the blood, and facilitate its passage through the bowels. The presence of bile is indispensable to perfect digestion. We presume it to be of great consequence in the animal economy, from the immense size of the organ, or machine employed to prepare it. It is the duty of the liver to prepare the bile. The stomach is placed in the left upper side of the abdomen, and partly under the short ribs. The liver occupies the right side of the top of the abdomen, and is divided into several lobes or divisions, lying partly under the short ribs; and a flap of it extends on the left side, considerably upon the stomach. The liver weighs a number of pounds, say from five to ten times as much as the empty stomach; it is by far the heaviest organ of the interior of the body.

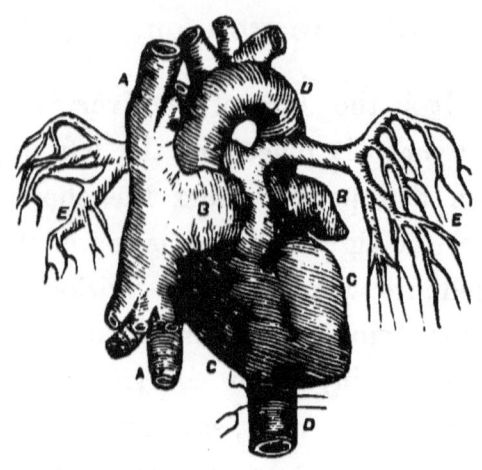

The Heart and its Blood Vessels.

CHAPTER XXIII.

THE HEART.

The heart and adjoining vessels are as follows:

The heart is composed of two auricles and two ventricles. The right auricle is joined at its posterior superior angle by the descending vena cava, and at its posterior inferior angle by the ascending vena cava; their columns of blood enter the auricle. Between the right auricle and ventricle there is a round hole for the passage of the blood, and this is called the ostium venosum. The ventriqularis dexter, which receives the blood from the right auricle, forms the anterior surface of the heart; it is separated from the left ventricle by a thick septum. There is an opening for the pulmonary artery above the ostium venosum. The pulmonary artery goes upward and backwards under the curvature of the aorta, and then divides into two trunks, one for each lung. The left auricle auriculis sinister posterior has an entrance into each of its angles for two pulmonary veins, two on each side, and, as in the right auricle, there is a hole about an inch in diameter, which communicates with the left ventricle. The left ventrical resembles an ovidal or conical body; the parieties, or walls, of this cavity are much thicker and stouter than the others, as it has the most laborious work to perform, but it decreases in thickness as it approaches the aorta. The heart is encased in a sack called the pericardium, and is covered on its sides by the placea or covering of the lungs; the pericardium covers the aorta up as high as the vessels proceeding from its arch. The coronary arteries arise from the trunk of the aorta. Veins bearing the same name follow in the course of the arteries. The nerves of the heart come from the cervical ganglion of the sympathetic nerve, and follow in the course of the arteries. While the circulation goes on, both auricles contract at the same instant, and the blood is thrown into the ventricles — the ventricles then contract and throw the blood into the aorta and pulmonary artery. From the curvature of the aorta, while it is crossing, the trachea vessels arise called the arteria innominata, the left primitive carotid and the left subclavian; the arteria innominata in ascending from right to left forms the right subclavian and the right primitive carotid; the left primitive carotid arises from the aorta. Just above the sternum and clavicle; the carotid is covered by the sterno-hyoid and thyroid muscles; the carotid having arrived as high as the os hyoides and thyroid cartillage divides into two large trunks: the internal carotid, which goes to the brain and the eye, and the external carotid, which is distributed upon the superficial parts of the head and the neck; the internal carotid extends from the larynx to the sella turnia, and ultimately penetrates into the cranium, through the carotid canal of the temporal bone, and sends off branches to various parts of the brain; the external carotid gives off branches to the superior thyroid and is distributed to the larynx and thyroid gland; the lingual artery also proceeds from this vessel, supplying the tonsils, palate, and epiglottis; it also communicates with the facial artery.

I have before referred to the fact, that consumption is often caused by irregular action of the heart, and by disease of the heart. The heart often has diseases of its own, independently of association or sympathy with any other organs; yet there is no organ of the whole body that is more influenced by the condition of other organs than the heart. The condition of the stomach powerfully influences the heart, and so does falling of the bowels, before referred to, and falling of the womb, and so does the condition of the lungs. The lungs, the stomach, the bowels, and the brain, may produce what seems to be heart disease when the heart is not at all diseased. The heart is often greatly affected by the condition of the walls of the chest itself. It is very often noticed that by stooping and leaning the shoulders heavily upon the chest, it is contracted at its base in front, and the breast-bone thrown flat down upon the heart, in this way injuring the heart, and leading to the opinion that there is disease of the heart, when there is no disease of it; but the walls of the chest have closed around it, and the heart cannot act. After forty years of age, and in a great many cases at an earlier period, the heart begins to enlarge in a multitude of persons, and, if the chest enlarges also, all is well; but if the chest does not enlarge, then the heart is compressed, and palpitation, suffocation of the heart, and apoplexy, may take place. From this fact is explained the reason why we have little heart disease until after the middle periods of life.

That heart diseases often arise from consumptive influences, I have verified in a great many cases. Knowing this, I have often ascertained the presence of heart disease in one or both parents, when I have found the children highly consumptive; yet nothing of consumption in any respect has shown itself in the parents. The treatment of heart disease, in a great many cases, is required to be the same as we find necessary in consumption; in fact, with a little modification, I treat many cases of heart disease the same as I do consumption, and often have the pleasure of entirely curing it, when all hope of life had fled. Of course, inhalants are not required if no cough exists.

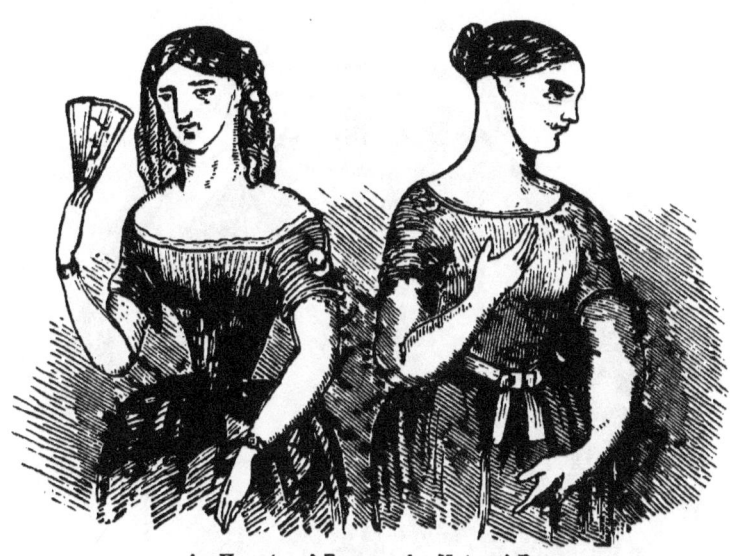

An Unnatural Form and a Natural Form.

CHAPTER XXIV.

TIGHT LACING.

A great deal has been said and written against the habit of tight lacing, or confining the waist, so as to make it very small. You will notice, by recalling what I have said, how pernicious and destructive lacing the chest must be to the lungs, the heart, the liver, and large bowels. It produces a broken constitution, and almost certain death to any or all who practice it. It is utterly subversive of symmetry, and is, in every point of view, decidedly vulgar. No person is now known to practice it, save the ignorant and the *would-be* fine and genteel. It must not be practiced if you would have health, elegance, or symmetry of person.

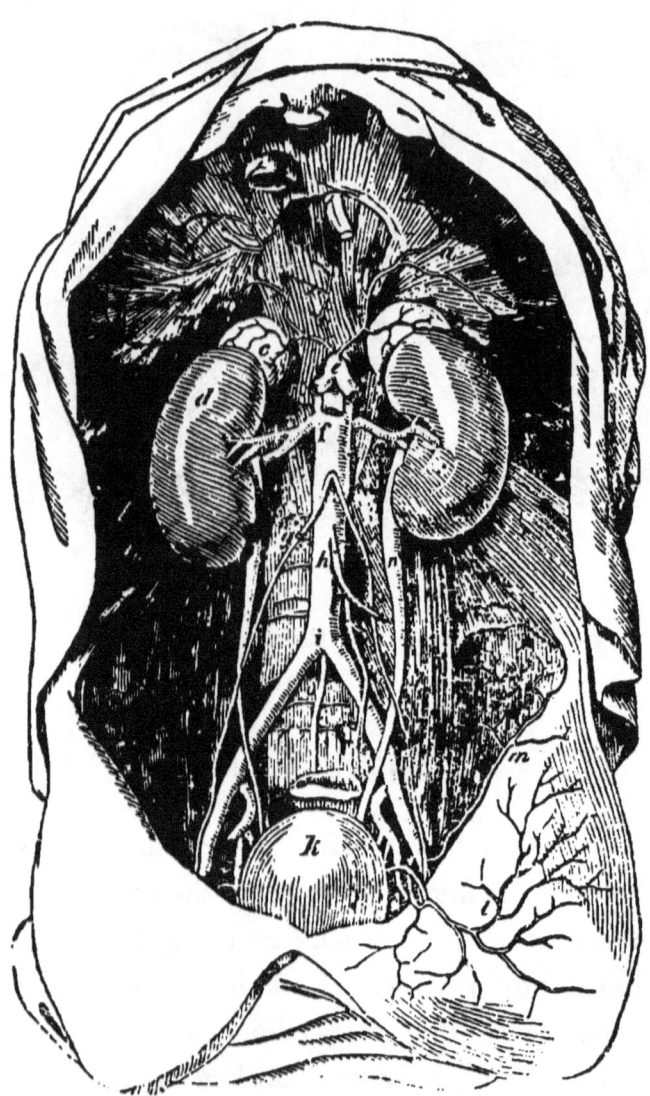

KIDNEYS, URETERS, &c.

A, the Midriff, or floor of the Lungs. *D D*, the Kidneys. *N N*, the Ureters, or pipes that carry the water from the Kidneys to the Bladder. *G O*, the Rectum. *K*, the Bladder. *E F H I*, the Aorta, &c.

CHAPTER XXV.

GRAVEL PRODUCED BY FALLING OF THE BOWELS, &c.

By looking at the plate on the preceding page you will see the position of the kidneys; each side of the spine, just above the point of the hips, and behind all the other contents of the abdomen. You will notice, also, two pipes that go, one from each kidney, forwards and downwards, behind the floating bowels, and down into the basket of the hips, to the back of each side of the bladder. These pipes, five to eight inches long, carry the water from the chamber of each kidney to the bladder. Now, then, when the floating bowels roll downwards, they often fall upon the pipes, and close them, more or less, so that the water is prevented from passing into the chambers of the bladder. This throws it back into the kidneys, and soon fills up the kidneys. The water usually has salts, and earths, and acids, &c., which it holds very lightly in solution. These salts, when the water stands any length of time, soon separate from it, and fall down. This you can daily see in the chamber vessels. These earths, in a short time will glue together, and form masses, more or less large, from the size of grains of fine sand, to lumps that weigh several ounces. At times all the walls of the chambers of the kidneys, and the pipes that carry the water from them to the bladder, are encrusted over with this sand. When this earthy matter is in the form of fine sand, it is called gravel. If it cements into masses larger than small peas, it is called stone. The pipes that carry the water from the kidneys to the bladder, are called the ureters; they have no popular name, that I have ever heard of. When the ureters are obstructed, and the water thrown back into the kidneys, its earliest effect is to cause great heat in the small of the back, and, at times, great soreness each side of the spine, just above the hip. Sometimes almost feeling as if in the hip, and even lameness in the hip will at times take place. If only one pipe is obstructed, one kidney only will be affected. Gravel is one of the most painful diseases to which we are liable. Sometimes pieces of stone will pass from the kidneys along the water-pipes to the bladder, and, if large, usually causing the most distressing and insufferable pain of which we are susceptible.

CHAPTER XXVI.

AIR AND VENTILATION.

TO MOTHERS.

We have only to contrast the blanched and feeble appearance of children inhabiting the dark and narrow streets of a crowded city, with the rosy freshness of those of the same classes residing on the suburbs or in the country, to obtain a pretty correct notion of the importance of a well selected locality. Considering the susceptibility of the influence of cold in early infancy, I need hardly add that a high and bleak situation, or one exposed to the full force of the north and east winds, is equally unfavorable and ought to be carefully avoided.

Cellars are damp and unhealthy. In selecting rooms for a nursery, those which have a southern exposure ought to be preferred. That a nursery ought also to be *large, easily warmed*, and *easily ventilated*, will, I think, be readily admitted; for, without such conditions, it is evidently impossible to surround an infant with that pure and renovating atmosphere which is indispensable to health.

In one respect, pure air is even more essential to the formation of good blood than supplies of proper food. The influence of the air we breathe *never ceases for a single moment of our lives,* while that of food recurs only at intervals. By night and by day, respiration goes on without a pause; and, every time we breathe, we take in an influence necessarily good or bad, according to the quality which surrounds us.

No wonder, then, that a cause, thus permanently in operation, should, after a lapse of time, produce great changes on the health; and no wonder that attention to the purity of the air we breathe should amply and surely reward the trouble we may bestow in procuring it. Accordingly, of all the injurious influences by which childhood is surrounded, few, indeed, operate more certainly or extensively than the constant breathing of a corrupt and vitiated air; and, on the contrary, few things have such an immediate and extensive effect in renovating the health of a feeble child, as change from a vitiated to a purer atmosphere.

Vitiated air and bad food are the two grand sources of that hydra-headed scourge of many countries—scrofulous diseases; and either of them, in a concentrated state, is sufficient to produce it, without the co-operation of the other; but when both are combined, as they often are among the poor in our larger towns, then scrofula in its worst form is the result. Accordingly, we can produce scrofula in the lower animals at will, simply by confining them in a vitiated atmosphere, and restricting them to an impoverished diet.

Scrofula, in one or other of its numerous forms, is acknowledged to be in Great Britain (and possibly in the United States) perhaps the most prevalent and fatal disease which afflicts the earlier years of life. It is the most usual cause of grandular obstructions, defective nutrition, affections of the joints, and other morbid conditions, which either give rise to, or greatly aggravate the danger of many other diseases—such as consumption, measles, hooping-cough, fever, teething, and convulsions; and in this way it proves fearfully destructive of life. But so powerful is the continued breathing of a cold, damp, and vitiated atmosphere in producing it, that where such a cause is allowed to operate, the most promising combination of other conditions will often prove insufficient to ward off the evil. Sir James Clark expresses the conviction that living in an impure atmosphere is even more influential in deteriorating health than defective food, and that the immense mortality among children reared in the work-houses, is ascribable even more to the former than to the latter cause.

So long ago as 1810, Mr. Richard Carmichael, of Dublin, in an excellent letter treatise on scrofula, drew the attention of the medical profession to this cause, and, on the strongest evidence, denounced the great impurity of the air in the Dublin house of industry as the grand cause of the excessive prevalence of scrofula among the children at the time he wrote. In one ward, measuring sixty feet by eighteen, and of very moderate height, there was *thirty-eight* beds, each containing *three* children, or 114 children in all. When the door was opened in the morning, the matron found the air insupportable, and, during the day, the children were either in the same ward, or crowded to the number of several hundred in a school-room. Keeping in mind the necessity of pure air to the formation of healthy and nutritive blood; we can scarcely feel surprised that scrofula was extremely prevalent under circumstance so calculated for its production.

When the weather is cold and damp, the windows ought never be thrown open till the children are removed, and the sun has been for some time above the horizon. The bedclothes ought to be turned down as soon as the child is taken up, and to be exposed to the air for several hours, that they may be entirely freed from the effluvia collected during the night. This point is, in general, too little attended to; the appearance of order and neatness being generally preferred to the real welfare of the child. While due care is taken to insure an adequate temperature, every approach to overheating must be scrupulously avoided.

CHAPTER XXVII.

SLEEP.

TO MOTHERS.

When the stomach is distended, and digestion just beginning, sleep is generally uneasy and disturbed. The infant, therefore, ought not to be put to rest immediately after a full meal. During the first month, it is true, he goes to sleep immediately after having the breast, but he sucks little at a time, and the milk is then so diluted as scarcely to require digestion; it is at a later period that the precaution becomes really important.

So much must always depend on individual constitution, health and management, that no fixed hours can be named at which the infant should be put to rest. If he sleeps tranquilly, and when awake is active and cheerful, and his various bodily functions are executed with regularity, we may rest assured that no great error has been committed, and that it is a matter of perfect indifference whether he sleeps an hour more or an hour less than another child of his own age. When, on the contrary, he sleeps heavily or uneasily, and when awake is either stupid or fretful, and his other functions are perverted, we may be certain that some error has been committed, and that he is either rocked to sleep immediately after a full meal, or otherwise mismanaged.

There are few things which distress an anxious mother or annoy an impatient nurse more than sleeplessness in her infant child, and there is nothing which both are so desirous to remove by the readiest means which present themselves. A healthy child, properly treated, and not unduly excited, will always be ready for sleep at the usual time; and, when it appears excited or restless, we may infer with certainty that some active cause has made it so, and should try to find it. If no adequate external cause can be discovered, we may infer with equal certainty that its health has in some way suffered, and that it is sleepless from being ill. In this case, the proper course is to seek professional advice, and to employ the means best adapted for the restoration of health, after which sleep will return as before.

From not attending to the true origin of the restlessness, however, and regarding it merely as a state troublesome to all parties; many mothers and nurses are in the habit of resorting immediately to laudanum, sedative drops, poppy-syrup, spirits, and other means of forcing sleep, without regard to their effects on the disease and on the system; and are quite satisfied if they succeed in inducing the appearance of slumber, no matter whether the reality be sleep, stupor or apoplectic oppression. The mischief done in this way is inconceivably great, and astonishment would be excited if it were generally known what quantities of quack "cordials," "anodynes," and even spirits are recklessly given with the view of producing quiet and sleep. In Germany, milk mixed with a decoction of poppy-heads is in common use for this purpose; Von Ammon mentions a case of a child, six months old, whose parents were delighted with the placid slumber induced by it, but in the morning were horrified to find the body stiff, and the extremities cold, the eyes turned up, and the surface covered with a cold sweat. Many an infant, the true cause of whose death was not always suspected even by the guilty person, has thus passed prematurely to its grave.

In infancy, as in adult age, it is highly conducive to health and sound sleep, that the night and bed clothes should be thoroughly purified by several hours exposure to the air every day, before the child is put to bed. The effect of perfectly fresh covering is soothing, and healthful in a high degree. The quantity of bedclothes ought to be quite sufficient to sustain the natural heat of the body, without being so great as to relax or excite perspiration; and for this reason a soft, yielding feather-bed is very objectionable, particularly in summer or in a warm room. In infancy, there is a natural tendency of blood to the head, and, where this is encouraged by warm caps, the consequences are often hurtful. The head, therefore, ought only to be slightly covered.

When the infant is habitually restless, bathe the whole surface with tepid water.

CHAPTER XXVIII.

DYSPEPSIA.

This is known to exist in some persons by a sensation of weight in the stomach after eating; in others, by a sour stomach; in others, heart-burn; in others, by great distress in the stomach after eating, taking place in a few minutes, or in one or two hours; in others, by a great deal of wind in the stomach; in others, by severe head-aches; in others, by a chronic diarrhœa, the food coming away unchanged; in others, the effects are chiefly evinced by pains in different parts of the body, more often in the left side, or from the breast-bone through to the back-bone, &c. In others, dyspepsia is manifested by great palpitation of the heart. In a vast many cases, true heart disease begins with dyspepsia; and in many others, what seems, by the great palpatation and stoppage of the heart, and irregular breathing, to be a genuine disease of the heart itself, is not so, but is caused by indigestion. Some, or all of the foregoing symptoms, and many more, such as cough, mentioned in another place, are found to exist in dyspepsia. I might mention sleeplessness, nervousness, beating of the heart on lying down in bed at night, often arise from indigestion. The effect of continued indigestion is, to reduce the strength, to take the color from the face, and, in many cases, to cause the face to become the color of a tallow candle. At other times, it causes great rushing of the blood to the head and face. It is the fruitful parent of skin diseases, or is intimately connected with them. If a good deal of bile comes into the stomach, it is apt to cause the skin of the neck, the forehead, &c., to become very thick and gross, and to break out in red pimples, greatly disfiguring the face, and utterly destroying the beauty of the complexion. I have only space to indicate to you a few of the articles of food that incline to dyspepsia, without having time to name many other causes of this disease. To have good digestion, the food should be eaten slowly, and well and perfectly chewed, or masticated. If the teeth of any one are bad, the food should be prepared in cooking, so as to require but little chewing, or mastication. Good digestion depends very much on our choice of food. It is utterly impossible to lay down rules of diet that do not find a great many exceptions in their application. We have several times had something like a fanaticism start up on the subject of diet. In these cases, it will be found that one man attempts to apply his experience to all mankind. Should his experience happen to be contrary to universal experience, he will be greatly disappointed in its good effects. For example, one has told us never to eat meat. On attempting to apply the rule of not eating meat to the general masses of men, it is found to fail, or, when attempted to be adopted, has produced the most disastrous results. It is most true that, what agrees with one may not agree with another. One can live on very light food, one requires very hearty food; one can be abstemious, others are destroyed by it; one can eat meat, one can leave it off. In all this, you must be directed by your own experience. In general, you should practice a wholesome carelessness about your food, eating a little of anything you please, unless you know it injures you. Eat enough, but never indulge in excess. I will mention one or two articles often used, that most generally have a bad effect upon the complexion, and are most usually injurious, especially if used before thirty years of age, or even at any period of life. Good fresh butter, not at all rancid, and eaten without being melted, is, in a vast many cases, and most usually, a very good article in the composition of our diet. But all the grease that is procured from lard, rancid butter, or animal oils, or gravies, is most injurious to the complexion.

I will inform you how it acts. Oils or fats, on being thrown into the stomach, cannot be digested by the juices of the stomach, as these incline to be acid, and will not digest them well. In order to do this, it is necessary to call bile into the stomach, which is a kind of soap; and grease, fats, &c., will not digest in the stomach, until bile joins and reduces them to a kind of soap, so that much greasy food for ladies will be found to make them bilious, and produce more or less of dyspepsia, in one or other of its forms. Now, we find that grease or rancid butter, or at least melted butter, enters very largely into the composition of pie-crust, and all forms of pastry, and into some kinds of cake, &c. These injuriously affect the stomach. This is the case with fat food, that is highly seasoned, as pork, sausages, &c. So that a lady who would have a fine complexion, and good digestion, must avoid fat meats, rich fat gravies, highly seasoned fat hashed meats, pastry, and every species of diet where fat enters largely into the preparation. Again, new bread, and all hot bread, will be found hard to digest, and, as a general rule, should be avoided. Coffee is very generally used, and by some persons who attain to considerable age, and speak of it in raptures; yet, from the experience of many thousand dyspeptics, who have consulted me, I find no article of diet more generally injurious to the dyspeptic, than coffee. Its effects are almost universally, if much drank, to produce dyspepsia, acidity, nervousness, palpitation of the heart, head-aches, dizziness, costiveness, covering the face with pimples, and making the skin of the face thick yellow, coarse, and repulsive, destroying both rose and lily. Its earliest effect is to destroy the complexion, produce sallowness, and great biliousness, when no injury whatever is suspected. It inclines to produce in those predisposed to them, bleeding lungs, and to develope scrofula and skin diseases. Children should never taste it, except at long intervals, say once a year or month. Black tea in moderation, milk, and also water, or milk and water, are good articles for drink. Late suppers should be avoided. Our food should never be taken much, if any, warmer than new milk.

CHAPTER XXIX.

ERYSIPELAS.

Erysipelas is known in Scotland as St. Anthony's Fire or Rose, an inflammation of the skin characterized by redness, swelling, and burning pain, commonly spreading from a central point, and sometimes affecting the subcutaneous cellular tissue. Idiopathic erysipelas almost invariably attacks the face; frequently it is preceded by loss of appetite, languor, headache, chilliness, and frequency of pulse; a spot now makes its appearance, commonly on one side of the nose, of a deep red color, swollen, firm, and shining, and is the seat of a burning, tingling pain. The disease gradually extends often until the whole of the face and hairy scalp have been affected, but it is exceedingly rare for it to pass upon the trunk. Often, while still advancing in one direction, the part originally affected is restored to its normal condition. Commonly large irregular vesicles filled with serum, precisely similar to those produced by a scald, make their appearance on the inflamed skin. The pulse is frequent, there is total loss of appetite, headache, prostration, restlessness, and sleeplessness, and commonly, particularly at night, more or less delirium is present. The complaint runs its course in about a week, and the general symptoms ordinarily abate somewhat before any decline is noticed in the local inflammation. In itself erysipelas of the face is ordinarily unattended with danger; but where it occurs in the course of other and exhausting diseases, it adds much to the gravity of the prognosis. In fatal cases the delirium is apt gradually to lapse into coma. Erysipelas is subject to epidemic influences; in certain seasons it is exceedingly prevalent, while in others it is rarely seen. The attack is favored by overcrowding and deficient ventilation. Hospitals, particularly in the spring of the year, are infested with it. Certain unhealthy states of the system predispose strongly to the disease, and an unwholesome diet and the abuse of alcoholic stimulants are commonly cited among its causes. We have seen that simple erysipelas is rarely fatal; consequently recoveries are common under a great variety of treatment. Usually it requires nothing more than to move the bowels by a mild laxative, and afterward to support the system by the administration of nutriment, and if necessary the use of simple medicines. Systematic writers make a separate variety of the erysipelas of new-born children; it presents no peculiarity, however, except its greater gravity, in common with other diseases, in such delicate organisms. When erysipelas of the abdomen occurs in new-born children, it commonly has its point of origin in the recently divided umbilical cord. In some cases erysipelas, arising generally from some injury or excoriation, shows a tendency to advance in one direction while it passes away in another (*erysipelas ambulans*); in this manner it may pass in turn over almost every part of the surface.

In phlegmonous erysipelas the precursory symptoms are more constant and severe, the pain more violent, the prostration greater; the redness is most strongly marked along the trunks of the lymphatic vessels, and the lymphatic glands are swollen; the swelling of the skin is more considerable, it soon assumes a pasty consistence, and pits strongly on pressure. As the disease advances, the pain subsides, the redness is diminished, and fluctuation becomes evident; if left to itself, the skin, gradually thinned and distended, sloughs over a larger or smaller space, and pus mingled with shreds of dead cellular tissue is discharged. The disease indeed seems often to be in the cellular tissue rather than in the skin, and sometimes the cellular tissue throughout a limb appears to be affected. It is a disease of great severity, and, when extensive, often proves fatal under the best treatment. In its treatment, the same general principles apply as in simple erysipelas. The patient's strength should be supported by a nutritious diet, and tonics and stimulants must often be freely administered. Early in the disease the skin should be freely divided down into the cellular tissue, to relieve the constriction of the parts and afford an early opening to the discharges.

CHAPTER XXX.

DROPSY.

Dropsy is a collection of serous fluid occurring in one or more of the closed cavities of the body or in the cellular tissues, independent of inflammation. Inflammations of serous membranes, pleurisy, pericarditis, peritonitis, &c., are often attended with copious effusion; but the effusion here depends immediately upon the inflammation, and consists of the liquor sanguinis, not of serum alone. Dropsy is a symptom and not a disease, and is caused either by pressure exerted upon some part or the whole of the venous system, or by an altered state of the blood. In the vast majority of cases dropsy depends upon disease of the liver, the heart, or the kidneys. From the peculiarity of the hepatic circulation, when cirrhosis of the liver exists, the venous system of all the abdominal viscera becomes congested, and that congestion finally relieves itself by an effusion of serum into the sac of the peritoneum. In this way the swelling in ascites, dependent upon cirrhosis, begins in the abdomen, and the legs only become swollen secondarily.

A scirrhus or other tumor by which the vena portæ is compressed produces dropsy exactly in the same manner as cirrhosis. When there is disease of the heart, that organ has more or less difficulty in emptying itself of the blood which is thrown into it; the difficulty commonly commences at the left side of the heart, and congestion of the lungs is a consequence; finally the right side becomes affected, there is congestion of the general venous system, and swelling takes place in the more dependent parts of the body; the great cavities, the abdomen and the chest, are afterward involved, and the dropsy becomes general. In Bright's disease the cause of the dropsy is probably to be sought in the deteriorated character of the blood; in many cases disease of the heart is added to the affection of the kidneys, and increases the tendency to dropsy. Chlorosis, severe hemorrhages, any cachexia by which the character of the blood is greatly altered, are apt to be attended with more or less serous effusion into the cellular tissue.

(See illustration, pp. 104.)

CHAPTER XXXI.

SPINAL DISEASES; PAIN IN THE SIDE; BEDS, AND LYING IN BEDS, &c.

Spinal diseases often lead to diseased lungs, by the great debility they produce. This debility preventing a full free exercise and expansion of the lungs. The ancient writers on the lungs and consumption make a consumption of the back or spine. A vast many persons allow pain to continue a long time in the spine, between the shoulders, in the neck, and particularly in the lowest portions of the back-bone, hips, and extreme end of the back-bone; sometimes attended with heat, at other times not; sometimes tender to the touch, at other times a cold spot, &c.; curvatures of the spine, &c. In a vast many cases, and probably quite a large majority of the cases, there is no actual disease of the spine; but those pains originate from humor, loss of symmetry, rheumatism, &c.

From whatever cause produced, the effect is very injurious upon all the general functions of the system, and should receive early attention.

PAIN IN THE SIDE.

Pain in the side, or its cause, often by organic changes, or by producing inability or an indisposition to expand the chest, will at last injure the lungs in many cases, and should not be allowed but should be cured.

Luxurious feather or down beds should be avoided, as they greatly tend to effeminate the system and reduce the strength. For this reason beds should be elastic, but rather firm and hard; straw beds, hair mattresses, these on a feather bed are well; a most excellent mattress is made by combing out the husks or shuck that cover the ears of Indian corn.

Cold sleeping rooms are in general best, especially for persons in health; they should never be much heated for any person, but all should be comfortably warm in bed.

CHAPTER XXXII.

CLIMATE.

Many consumptives think they would enjoy perfect exemption, if they could reside in a hot climate. No mistake is greater than this; a hot climate, as a general rule, is not usually of much value; the effect of a hot climate is to debilitate and effeminate the system, and to predispose to consumption; hence, consumption is common in all the West Indies, and in all hot countries amongst the natives, and long residents. No climate is worse to a consumptive than where his disease originated; any change with him is for the better; going from the sea-board to the western country, avoiding a residence on the shores of great bodies of water. The new inland countries are the best; changing from the sea shores to the interior, even if not more than forty miles back. Removing from the mountains to the valleys, and from the valleys to the mountains, especially in summer, is most favorable; avoid locations where there is great prevalence of damp changeable weather. Consumption is as prevalent in any city of Cuba, as it is at Archangel, on the frozen ocean.

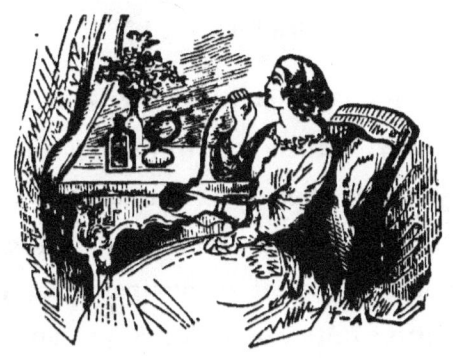

CHAPTER XXXIII.

TREATMENT OF DISEASE OF THE LUNGS AND AIR PASSAGES, BY THE INHALATION OF COLD AND WARM MEDICATED VAPORS.

For the last eighteen years, since I have been practicing as a specialist, for successfully treating and curing pulmonary consumption, and the various modern diseases of more refined and civilized life pertaining to the larynx, trachea and bronchia, I have been consulted by many thousands of invalids; many of whom were induced to adopt my treatment, either from their extreme suffering or their own good sense and moral independence, for in every case it was in extreme opposition to their family physician or medical attendants, who, after dosing drugs into the stomach until the whole system revolted longer to receive such nauseating potions, they were then greeted as the last consoling hope—that their case was one of incurable consumption, and it was folly to expect either relief or cure! This was the condition under which my patients applied and adopted treatment—given up to an inevitable doom, in one case even by five physicians. At this present time this very patient, thus consigned in the bloom of life to an early grave, has recovered, and being restored to good health and strength, is now able to enjoy the society of her family and friends, and mingle again in the pleasures of life.

I mention this case as being a specimen only of nearly all that daily apply to me. They have in many instances been doctored for years by allopathic physicians, who seem insane on the one idea that God made the human stomach for no other purpose than for receiving nauseous, poisonous and debilitating drugs, and after the patient is nearly worn out, the only consolation is that their case is hopelessly incurable, and when Inhalation has been suggested by the patient as the only ray of hope, they have been confronted by their physicians that it was only a system of humbugery and quackery—not having magnanimity of soul sufficient to recommend them to test its efficacy by a fair trial.

The profession which I feel proud to make my calling

—to the study and investigation of which I have spent the energies of my system, and the best portion of my days—is too noble and humane to shield anything that is narrow, exclusive, ignoble, or intolerant. I feel above that grade that seek to elevate themselves at the expense of calumny and persecution of a professional brother.

To those who will be pleased to call on me, professionally, they will find that I do not conceal from an honest and candid enquirer, any views pertaining to my peculiar mode of practice, and will extend to them all the privileges and civilities that should characterize the medical ethics of an enlightened faculty and a free republic.

For my own part, I shall feel secure in the high and laudable position I have taken, in bringing to the rescue of so many lives as are now going down to the grave, without any means being offered on the part of the old school physicians, so valuable a discovery as medicated inhalations, which bids fair to conquer its fatality, while its consolatory influence elicits from those subjects who had but to look to futurity involved in gloom and darkness, expressions of thankfulness and gratitude for their recovery, which will serve to cheer me during my earthly pilgrimage, and extend its cheering influence beyond the portals of the tomb.

CHAPTER XXXIV.

INHALANTS.

I use different Inhalants, which I prepare according to the requirements of each patient, and which are made from some of the following medicines, viz:

Iodine, Conium, Oxygen, Hydrogen, Nitrogen, Nitrous Gas, a great variety of Gums and Balsamic Resins, Vapor of boiling Tar, Hydrocyanic Acid, Camphor, Ammonia, Balsam Tolu, Naphtha, Chlorine, Hyoscyamus, Lactuca, Belladonna, Digitalic, Colchicum a great variety of Balsamic Herbs, Galbanum, Vapor of Vinegar, Nitre, Strammonium, Lobelia, Inflata, Ipecacuanha, Alcohol, Hydriodate of Potassa, Storax, Marshmallows, Rose Water, a great variety of Emollient and Narcotic Herbs, &c.

Pages 173-176 missing

6. *Combativeness*—Resistence, self-protection; spirit of opposition, resolution; disposition to brave danger.

7. *Destructiveness*—Executiveness, indignation, irritability, a destroying and pain-causing disposition; energy.

8. *Alimentativeness*—Appetite, desire of nutrition, sense of hunger, and capacity to enjoy food and drink.

9. *Acquisitiveness*—Desire to acquire and possess property, as such; its exercise tends to frugality and industry.

10. *Secretiveness*—Sense of secresy, concealment, cunning, evasion; disguising one's real sentiments and plans.

11. *Cautiousness*—Sense of danger: apprehension, delay, regard for present and future safety; fear, dread of results.

12. *Approbativeness*—Sense of character and appearance; desire to please, love of praise and popularity; vanity.

13. *Self-Esteem*—Self-regard; pride, independence, dignity; love of power and distinction; self-reliance.

14. *Firmness*—Decision, will, perseverance, stability, determination of purpose; unwillingness to yield.

15. *Conscientiousness*—Sense of moral obligation; regard for truth and justice; contrition, integrity, honesty, &c.

C. *Circumspection*—Sense of discretion, consistency, uniformity, and balancing power–[not fully established.]

16. *Hope* — Sense of immortality, and of the future; anticipation, expectation; looking forward for future results.

17. *Marvelousness* — Credulity; sense of the spiritual and supernatural; belief in invisible agency; faith, curiosity.

18. *Veneration* — Sense of greatness, adoration, respect for superiority, authority, and deference to age or antiquity.

19. *Benevolence* — Munificence, sympathy, disinterestedness, and desire to promote the happiness of others.

20. *Constructiveness* — Sense of mechanism, manual dexterity, contrivance, ingenuity, and skill.

21. *Ideality* — Sense of perfection; delicacy, taste, refinement, appreciation of the beautiful in nature and art.

B. *Sublimity* — Sense of the vast, the grand and the sublime in nature; love of the highest kinds of composition.

22. *Imitation* — Powers of representation, imitation, and adaptation; versatility of action; and ability to mimic others.

23. *Mirthfullness* — Perception of the absurd and ridiculous; gaiety, levity, playfulness, and buffoonery.

24. *Individuality* — Power to identify individual objects; observation of details; desire to be an eye-witness.

25. *Form* — Sense of shape, likeness, expression, and outline; memory of countenances and configuration.

26. *Size* — Sense of proportion, magnitude, equality, and relation of outlines; exactitude.

27. *Weight* — Sense of gravity; power to balance, and apply the laws of gravity in machinery and muscular motion.

28. *Color* — Sense of colors; their beauty, arrangement, and harmony in nature and painting.

29. *Order* — Sense of, and desire for convenience and arrangement; neatness, perception of general economy.

30. *Calculation* — Perception of numbers, and their relations; numerical computations.

31. *Locality* — Sense of place, position, and direction; memory of objects by location; desire to travel, see places, &c.

32. *Eventuality* — Sense of action, events, phenomena, statistical knowledge; memory of facts; love of narrative.

33. *Time* — Sense of chronology, of duration, of passing time; when, and how long; equality in step and beat in music.

34. *Tune* — Perception of sound, of melody, of proper emphasis, and modulation of the voice; ability to compose music.

35. *Language* — Sense of words or signs to com-

municate ideas; ability to talk; memory of names and words.

36. *Causality* — Sense of cause and effect; power of abstract thought; penetration, planning, invention, originality.

37. *Comparison* — Sense of resemblance, of analogies, similies, and power of analysis; association, comparison, &c.

MESMERISM.

A few remarks on that functional state of the nervous system, termed Mesmerism, may not be irrevalent to add in this treatise. It is called by some animal or human magnetism. It was known to the ancients, and has been revived by the moderns, particularly in the last century by Dr. Frederick Antony Mesmer, of France, from whom it has derived its name. Travellers in eastern countries describe paintings found in the temples of Thebes and other ancient cities which represent persons in a sleeping posture, while others are making passes over them. The priests of Chaldea, of Nineveh, of Babylon, of Judea, and Jerusalem, and the priests and physicians of ancient Greece and Rome practised magnetism in their temples and in the healing art, long before the Christian era. "Aristotle informs us that Thales, who lived six hundred years before Christ, ascribed the curative properties in the magnet to a soul with which he supposed it to be endowed, and without which he also supposed no kind of motion could take place." Pliny also affirms the magnet to be useful in curing diseases of the eyes, scalds, and burns; and Celsus, a philosopher of the first century after Christ, speaks of a physician by the name of Asclepiades, who soothed the ravings of the insane by manipulations, and he adds that his manual operations, when continued for some time, produce a degree of sleep or lethargy. Under the name of "neurology," attempts have been made in this country to put a new dress upon it, and to bring it before the public with new features, and to connect with it some new discoveries; but it remains to be what it has ever been, the principal difference being only different modes of illustration.

Of the nature of this mysterious principle or agent, we know but little, but of its effects on the system we are quite familiar; and it can be practised and demonstrated easily by any one a little acquainted with the method of operating upon those termed "impressible subjects." After repeated passes of the hand from the head downwards nearly in contact with the body, the subject falls into a mesmeric sleep, formerly called the *crisis*, in which the outward senses, particularly the sight, are apparently closed, and the interior or inward senses, are capable of seeing and describing objects not otherwise visible—as internal diseases, reading when blindfolded, &c. The body sometimes becomes fixed as in a trance, and is insensible to pain, so that even surgical operations have been performed in a magnetic sleep without causing distress.

A limb having been mesmerized, becomes stiff and almost immovable, and may be made to adhere firmly to the head, so that it cannot be forced off until the fluid has become withdrawn. The will of the person magnetized appears to be completely under the direction of the magnetizer. In this condition, if any of the phrenological organs be magnetized, it developes their peculiar character, and the subject involuntarily exercises them preternaturally; for instance, *combativeness*, which arouses the pugnacious or fighting propensities; if *amativeness*, the subject make loves to the operator. Some who make extravagant if not visionary pretensions to magnetism, asserts that by putting certain agents into the hand, such as Capsicum, Antimony, &c., their effects will be left upon the system; and no doubt those who have the organ of *marvelousness* largely developed suppose that some such effect is produced, with other strange fancies.

The question naturally arises, how far is it useful? This remains yet to be shown. Some attach great remedial power to magnetism, and, no doubt, in some cases, it exerts an influence, and may have proved useful; but as yet nothing very definite or certain has been established that we can rely upon. It would appear that those termed " clairvoyants " are able to detect diseases, but most of them are unable to prescribe successfully, as I have proved in my practice. How far this agent will be more fully developed remains to be seen. But probably much greater light will be thrown upon it by future investigations. Without doubt all the phenomena are to be referred to natural causes, and and not to superhuman or satanic agency, as has been supposed.

Some err, if not degrade themselves, by the false and visionary ideas they attach to magnetism. They make it their "hobby," and much of their ideality is associated with its wonderful effects on the system. To listen to them, we would suppose that their claims to discoveries were superior to all others. This manifests a peculiar state of mind bordering on *monomania*, and the healing art at least will not be much indebted to such for improvements.

The subject of animal magnetism now excites considerable interest in England and India, and some experiments have been made which illustrate very clearly its singular effects upon the system. Institutions and periodicals have been established to promote it, particularly among the poor, as a medical agent. A mesmeric infirmary has been established for the poor in Dublin, and one in *Madras*, in *India*, called the *Electic* Mesmeric Hospital. The British Government has appointed a committee to investigate its merits. The resident surgeon has reported several operations performed on native patients for large tumors, which were removed without pain, in the *mesmeric trance*, weighing from thirty to a hundred pounds. Dr. Esdaile, one of the surgeons of the Institutions in India, closes the report on the effects of mesmerism in the following language:—

"From the foregoing facts, I consider myself entitled to say that it has been demonstrated that patients in the mesmeric trance may be insensible to,

1st, The loudest noises.
2d, Painful picking and pinching.
3d, The cutting of inflamed parts.
4th, The application of nitric acid to raw surfaces.
5th, The racking of the electro-magnetic machine.
6th, The most painful surgical operation; and yet be aroused into full consciousness by the exposure of the naked bodies for a few minutes to the cold air."

APPENDIX.

TOBACCO; ITS ACTION ON THE HEALTH, AND ITS INFLUENCE ON THE MORALS AND INTELLIGENCE OF MAN.

With tobacco the savage endures hunger, thirst, and all atmospheric vicissitudes more courageously; the slave bears more patiently servitude, misery, &c. Among men who call themselves civilized, its assistance is often invoked against *ennui* and melancholy; it relieves sometimes the torments of disappointment of hopes or ambition, and contributes to console, in certain cases, the unfortunate victims of injustice; and enables lazy people to while away a dull hour in mental vacancy.

This is certainly a brilliant apology for the use of tobacco; but without comparing ourselves to those tribes of savages, droves of slaves, and lazy people, to whom this weed appears to render such signal services, will we not be permitted to say to Dr. Chamberet, that the remedy he extols to us so highly, is often worse than our complaints.

That the plant momentarily elevates the ideas, or at least withdraws them for some instants from their ordinary course, to be succeeded by a kind of stupidity, or apathy, to which many individuals are inclined, we do not deny; but also, like other errors and deplorable habits, do not many disorders and vicious inclinations follow in their train?

Most assuredly.

And when a person commences the use of it, is there any guarantee that he will use it moderately?

Evidently not, for unfortunately, he is as susceptible of the abuse of it, as of all joys by irritation; of these we will enumerate the game, strong liquors, the passions, &c.; and, as soon as a snuff-box is offered to him or he smells the smoke of a cigar or pipe, the demon tobacco, that never ceases to tempt him, will not permit him to rest until he has taken one pinch or smoked one cigar.

Suppose we admit — although we were tempted every day, every hour, every instant—we possess sufficient self-control and moral courage, as not to allow the poison time enough to produce its hurtful action; we ask, how many smokers, snuffers and chewers, despite the counsels of hygiene and of common sense, do we not see consume tobacco until they have fallen into a state of stupor and imbecility?

Besides, if, as is commonly written, the action of tobacco depends upon constitutional dispositions and hygienic conditions of the systems of the persons who use it, and the different quantities employed, how can you dare say that you do not dread its hurtful influence?

Behold that young and handsome lady who has so many admiring friends, and who, to drive away the *ennui* that darkens her brow, or obscures her mind, makes, at the instigation of her husband, the acquisition of a snuff-box, promising herself to take only one or two pinches of snuff daily. Her sense of smell is at first keenly excited, and as the powder exercises a gentle and slight titilation of the mucous membrane of the nose, as the mirror of her eyes glisten with silvery tears, and as she feels the dreaded *ennui* that besets her disappear, she opens again, and again, the fatal box; the habit of snuffing has already taken root in her nose, and if you should meet her some time afterward, you easily recognize her by the odor of tobacco that her breath spreads around her, by her dirty handkerchief and dress, by her nasal voice, by her dejected spirits, by her gaping mouth, by her nose plugged up with a black crust; and if she gestures in your presence, it will only be to cast her fingers unceasingly into her snuff-box, as if she had only preserved the instinct for that mechanical action.

Behold, on the other hand, that young man who has received, at birth, the most precious gifts that Providence accords to human nature, intelligence and health.

During the happy days of his scholastic struggles, he has gained the most beautiful victories, and his professors, happy to crown him with the laurels he so justly merits, applaud him for his success, predicting that he will take a stand in the highest ranks of society. Proud of all these flattering omens, and of the beautiful prism through which he beholds in such glittering colors the happy future, his mind, in which the germs of genius have been sown with the hand of God, expands every instant as it dives into the inexhaustible source of all the human sciences; but, melancholy to say, the day will come also, when the door of the orgies will be opened to him, and as nothing is more beautiful to the brilliant imagination of an impulsive youth, in a night of debauchery, than to see the sparkling gas of the champagne unite with the clouds of smoke that curl above his head, he will seize, for the first time in his life, a *cigar*; he will dirty his lips with its impure juice without for once thinking that a poison is concealed in the pleasure that he partakes of—a pleasure always renewed by its ashes, to lead continually to new desires and to new joys.

Oh, the poisonous *weed!* Though it makes him sick and loathe it the first time, it tempts him again, and as he " never surrenders," the magnanimous youth resolves to try and gain another victory. He smokes, and smokes again; and if one or two cigars surfice him to-day, in a month he will smoke three, four, or half a dozen per day, and in less than six months he sucks the nauseous pipe; a thousand emotions will come then to lend him the charm of their seducing and deceitful reveries; then, an epoch will arrive when his soul, which had always been so calm and so happy, will awaken with a start—a shudder, as if it felt the breath of an ardent passion pass over it. Yes, he is a confirmed smoker.

Follow now this young man into the world, and soon, be well assured, you will see him trembling in a manner, as his mouth emits, like the crater of Vesuvius, those streams of smoke which conceal the borders of the gulf in which, sooner or later, his physical forces and moral faculties will be found to be extinguished.

Though his temperament may be bilious, nervous, sanguineous, or phlegmatic, yet a multitude of general disorders will not be long in coming to be grafted upon it by the deplorable habit he has contracted. At first, he complains of a slight headache; he desires much to study, but the pain is stronger than his will; then, as his muscles have already lost a part of their power from the secondary effects of the narcotic which has congested his brain, he throws himself carelessly and lazily in an arm-chair, whilst his head, obeying its own weight, rolls like an inert ball over his shoulders, and his heavy eyelashes involuntarily close, and he in vain endeavors to open them; the poison that his system has absorbed paralyzes all his efforts. Stretching, and yawning, and sighs, spring blusteringly from the oppressed chest; his automatic movements stiffen momentarily his body; his trembling hands are borne upon his eyes to try and raise the thick veil that obscures his vision; finally, fearing not to be able to escape the arms of Morpheus open to receive him, he lays aside his book, to go and ask of his *idol* tobacco for a *little distraction*. Seizing a fresh sugar, he exclaims, "I will study to-morrow ;" but on to-morrow he is nauseated and desires to vomit, for it is necessary to bear in mind that tobacco, in stupefying the brain, hinders it from reacting on the stomach; this later organ not receiving its natural stimulus as usual, becomes inactive; the vital energy of this organ is soon destroyed, and the loss of appetite is manifested; and as, above all things, it is necessary to eat to enable the mind to elaborate whatever is presented to it, this young man, who closed his book yesterday, from drowsiness, refuses to-day all kinds of food, in consequence of the disgust which it creates.

Here are, then, two important organs presiding essentially over the fundamental acts of life, which we suddenly found enchanged, or singularly modied by tobacco.

Tobacco has the property of diminishing hunger. Ramazini says that many tnavellers have assured him that tobacco chewed or smoked drives away the appetite, and that one can travel much longer without being oppressed with hunger.

Van Helmont says the same thing; he contended that tobacco appeased hunger, not by satisfying it, but by destroying the sensation, and by diminishing the activity of the other functions.

Ramazini adds, he has often observed smokers and chewers without an appetite, as well as great wine-drinkers, because their usage enervates the action of the stomach.

Plempius likewise remarks, that tobacco diminishes the sense of hunger, but gives another reason in explanation of the phenomena; he believes that by the abundance of serum or saliva which flows into the stomach, and fills more or less this viscera, that the sense of hunger is appeased in consequence of its absorption, and not by its enervation or numbness.

But this is nothing; the habit of smoking will become so confirmed with him, that he will come to experience only a single pleasure, that of puffing and absorbing tobacco smoke every moment.

But this estacy of the senses, this continual enervation, in discarding from his mind the *ennui* that besets it, causes him almost to forget his duties. Again, this being an acquired habit, diverts necessarily the desires from their direct course, and, as a desire, as soon as satisfied, calls up another, the habit of smoking engenders a number of habits, the more unfortunate, too, in a manner, as he advances in life.

Do you not see already, there is no tobacco too strong for him? What will he do? Ah! my God! Since this poison has commenced to brutalize him, why will he go and drown his remorse, and exhaust the slight strength that remains with him with beer, wine or alcohol? From this moment, the wisest counsels, and the strongest arguments that can be produced, will not turn him from his vicious inclinations; he will be seen day and night to abandon his studies, and leave his family, to visit the smoking-rooms and drinking establishments, and swell the crowd of loafers, the best portion of whose lives are spent in contact with the cigar, the pipe, and the glass.

Let us stop here and close the picture. However, if after this young man has indulged in his favorite habits of smoking and chewing, and drinking spirituous liquors, for some years, we should chance to obtain a view of his exterior person, and dive into the recesses of his organization, what disorders will we not behold there? His face, with pallor and sadness confounded, indicates a state of suffering; his muscles, formerly so strong, and so vigorous, now flabby and shriveled, are effaced beneath a tarnished skin; his legs tremble as he moves, for the marasmus, in devouring by degrees the mass of cellular tissue which covers his members, has dried up many of the streams of his material life. If we pass from his physical to his intellectual faculties, to interrogate them, we will find in place of that intelligence which was so rich and brilliantly announced, a short time previous, not idiocy, if you wish, but a state of vacancy and stupidity such that, if some day, in meeting him, you take a fancy to ask him only to call your name, with whom he has been united in the ties of friendship from his infancy, you will see him hesitate a long while before pronouncing it.

It is lamentable to relate, but his memory, imitating in this particular the smoke of the thousands of cigars that he has consumed, has finished, like their fumes, by disappearing and vanishing in the air.

Thus, grace to this unfortunate present, which originating in the new world, has spread over the old world, here is a young man (and thousands can testify to the same thing), born to shine some day, at the head of literature, of the sciences, in the legislative halls, or in the army of his country, who has become to celebrate or acquire no other glory than that of having *culotter* pipes! He has sacrificed his health and beautiful prospects at the altar of his *idol*—the *demon tobacco*. How is it to be expected that an organization, which has not sufficient vigor to contend against the deteriorating influence of a weed so injurious to the human constitution, can be developed, and gain the strength which it requires, whilst habituating itself daily to the contact of such a poison?

Look at the people in the East, formerly so powerful, now so weak and extremely degraded, and tell us if they do not owe a part of their ignorance and degradation to this vice,—so fashionable among us! Tobacco increases the inclination that most men have to idleness, by destroying the ideas of remorse, which complete inaction or laziness never fails to give rise. It dissolves family circles, so much cherished by decent men, from which the men and young bucks escape, to go and smoke, and chew, and spit.

Just peep behind the curtains of the smoking-rooms of the United States, England, Holland, Belgium, Spain, France, Italy, &c., and see their inmates with shallow heads, and vacant minds, happy to be plunged in a sea of amber and liquor, and enveloped in a fog of smoke, which seems to afford them more solid joys than the pleasures of ladies' society, and the sweets of the domestic fireside.

Is it not most astonishing, that civilized and decent men should lead such lives? It is well known, that during the manufacture of tobacco, there arises from the plant such strong and such unhealthy dust, as to cause great inconvenience to those engaged in the labor.

All writers on the subject describe the laborers as generally emaciated, tarnished, yellow, asthmatic, subject to colics, looseness, bloody flux, dyspepsia; but above all, to vertigo, headache, muscular twitchings, cramps, and more or less acute diseases of the chest, as we have frequent occasions to observe, either in the public walks, in the tobacco factories, or hospitals.

Thus, a substance so useless produces innumerable ills, and death even to those charged to prepare for others the most insignificant of pleasures.

There arises, indeed, particularly in summer, such quantities of subtile particles — dust — in tobacco factories, that the neighbors of them are much incommoded, and are frequently made sick at the stomach.

The horses employed turning the mills that grind and powder the tobacco, manifest the hurtful effects of the dust which surrounds them, by frequently agitating their heads, coughing, and snorting. The laborers suffer much from headache, vertigo, nausea, and loss of appetite, and continual looseness.

Those endemic diseases of which we have spoken, have spread with such violence among the people residing around and near tobacco factories, that in some countries, the wise precaution is adopted of establishing the factories outside of the towns; this precaution is particularly observed, at present, in France.

Remember now, that diseases do not always manifest themselves by phenomena—symptoms, so plain that it suffices for the most inexperienced eye to recognize them. There are poisons which, given in certain doses, and in certain forms, will kill as dead as if we were struck with lightning. Take now the same dose of this same medicine; but, before, study its action; as you have been so murderous, divide it into fiftieths and in hundredths of grains; then, if you wish to establish upon yourself a scale of comparison, take it into your stomach in the least possible form; take it daily, being careful to augment gradually the dose, and at the end of two or three months, you will be able to support a dose of poison, that, taken all at once, before commencing its use, would kill you instantaneously.

Let us go a little further. In graduating thus the doses of this substance, that bears death with it, when we take not the wise precaution to divide its force, and neutralize its effects, you may, perhaps, have experienced no ill effects from it; but put yourself every day, for six months, or a year, under the influence of the same preparation, and the time will come, be well assured, when your health, though good in appearance, will suffer seriously, and without your perceiving the hurtful blows that you have directed against it.

THE ORGANIC CHANGE WHICH TOBACCO PRODUCES IN THE NOSE.

We believe that certain snuffers stuff their nose with the vile poison until they blindly develop in that important organ the germs of a multitude of diseases, such as *inflammatory affections, lachrymal fistulas, polypuses, cancers, &c.*

We will now proceed to take a rapid sketch of each of these disorders.

NASAL CATARRH, COLD IN THE HEAD.

All authors consider snuff as the first and most frequent cause of cold in the head.

This affection consists, in the beginning, of a dryness, heat, redness, and swelling of the pituitary membrane, with shivering, sneezing, a sense of weight at the root of the nose, a dull, aching pain in the head, loss of smell, sometime itching of the nasal fossas, with stopping up of the nostrils, and a decided nasal voice; all the result of congestion of the mucous membrane of the parts. This membrane once congested, inflammation succeeds, and does not remain dry long; it becomes very soon the seat of an abundant, aqueous, colorless, ratty secretion, producing by its acrimony excoration of the upper lip, and angles of the nose themselves.

Most snuffers thus affected, fail not then to snuff more freely. Henceforth, the thicker the excreting matter becomes, the more they are led to praise the happy benefits of their remedy; they will refuse to renounce their remedy, without doubting, if a healthy person were to employ the same means, it would produce infallibly the same result — that is, the same *purgation*. The inflammation is sometimes most violent; the pain seems to be seated in the frontal sinuses, and is very acute, the head is heavy, and the teguments of the nose and cheeks become swollen, &c.

If, in spite of the suffering that the snuffer experiences, he continues as usual to take snuff, the malady progresses, and either forms abscesses in the maxillary fossas, that are very painful, but generally burst and discharges the thick purulent matter through the nostrils, or else becomes a true chronic catarrh; which consists in a very abundant nasal discharge, differing from the nasal mucous. This matter sometimes remains limpid, colorless, and without odor; sometimes it is thick, yellow, or green, and fœtid; sometimes, in fact, it is purulent; in this case there is ulceration of the pituitary membrane, an ulceration that has received the name of ozena.

OZENA.

This name is given to ulcers seated in the nostrils, from which issues a fœtid discharge, and persons affected with this repulsive disease, pass under the generic name of *punais* — one who has a *stinking nose*.

This affection commences, sometimes, among snuffers, with an intollerable stopping up of the nose, which is soon accompanied, and principally at the time the inflamed pituitary membrane passes to the state of ulceration, with headache that is exasperated at night. At other times they experience a dull, heavy, deep, itching, sensation; the nose swells and reddens; the voice changes; and if the ulcers are visible to the eye, they are seen covered with a grayish scab, or thick, brown, dry, muco-purulent crust, which falls off by degrees each time that the patient blows his nose hard, but fails not to form again soon after.

In fact it is unnecessary to say a loss of smell, or, at least, a very sensible diminution in this faculty of perceiving odors, is constantly remarked among those snuffers attacked with this repulsive and disgusting disease, against which the surgeon possesses but slight means to relieve, unless the patient renounces the habit of snuffing.

FISTULA LACHRYMALIS.

We have already remarked that the tears flow into the nasal fossas through two small canals extending from the inner angles of the eyelids and terminating in the nostrils, called lachrymal ducts; and added, that these two canals, like the nasal fossas, are lined with a mucous membrane.

These simple anatomical facts being premised, suppose the nostrils are highly inflamed for an instant by tobacco, what will happen? For however flat the nose may be from congenital effect, or from any other cause, the inflammation, in extending itself into these canals, will terminate, very likely, in obliterating them; and the tears, not being able to pass through these ducts, will accumulate in a sac, the walls of which will inflame in turn, and *fistula lachrymalis*, or false opening will soon appear, which will give exit to the tears and a puriform matter, that will run down the cheeks, and spoil the prettiest face. They are very troublesome to cure.

POLYPUS OF THE NASAL FOSSAS.

According to some authors this name originated in the fact that the polypus of the nose sends numerous roots into all the cavities or infractuosities of the nasal fossas, and constrains the respiration, in the same manner that polypus of the sea annoys fishermen with their long arms.

Whatever may be the origin of this name, we call thus commonly, the fleshy, fibrous, fungous excrescences, which can be developed upon all the mucous membranes, but which are more frequently observed in the interior of the nose.

The causes that produce polypus, says MM. Roche and Lanson, are sometimes unknown. Nevertheless, add they, they are so often seen to attack persons who are inveterate snuff-takers, that we are justified in concluding that a continual irritation of the pituitary membrane, is not, in many cases, foreign to their development.

A brief sketch of the symptoms of this frightful disease, we hope, will perhaps be the means of inducing some sufferers to abandon forever their snuff-box.

The patient complains first of a stopping up of the nostril, he breathes with difficulty with the affected nostril, he experiences the sensation of a soft foreign body in the nostril, and endeavors, by frequent blowing and sneezing, to get rid of it. The nostril soon becomes completely obstructed. The constraint occasioned to the respiration by the polypus is not always the same, nor constant; it is greater during humid than dry weather, and it sometimes happens that the patient feels completely relieved of it for sometime after having expelled from the nose a given quantity of limpid serum.

In the first case, the polypus seems to absorb and return its humidity to the air, like a sponge. In the second, its substance is torn, disgorged of serum, and contracts until the wound is cicatrized; it then retains again the serum it secretes. When polypuses arise near the posterior part of the nostril, they hang down in the throat; when they originate in the front part of the nostril, they compress the inferior orifice of the lrchrymal duct of which we have spoken, and misdirect the course of the tears, and if not, they do not occasion *lachrymal fistulas*, at least a continual flow of tears.

As soon as they have advanced toward the anterior and posterior openings of the nostrils, and filled them up, they penetrate the maxillary sinuses, dilate them, and perforate them to project toward the cheek, or in the mouth by the inferior wall of the orbit, push the eye from its cavity, and send, in fine, branches in the temporal fossas, and sometimes, even, to within the cavity of the cranium, pushing aside or perforating the bone.

Before such a picture, many snuffers may exclaim, they have snuffed tobacco for ten, twenty, or thirty years without ever experiencing the least signs of the affection we have described; but if you are well to-day, can you deny that you may not be sick to-morrow?

In conclusion, gentle reader, if you have perused our pages so far, you will perceive we have considered tobacco in relation to the physiological and toxicological phenomena which manifest themselves in those who use and abuse it. But its injurious action does not stop there.

It is evident, indeed, that if this plant has sufficient power to modify the intelligence, the sensibility, and volition to the degree to occasion in them disorders more or less serious, it must necessarily leave traces of its passage upon the parts with which it comes in immediate and almost continued contact.

Of course, a plant so *savory* should be presented to its numerous consumers in many different forms, to suit all their different tastes.

Such is the fact, tobacco is introduced into the nose in the form of powder, by snuffing; into the mouth, in powder by dipping, and in leaves by chewing; and more frequently, in fumes by smoking. It remains now to study its irritating action in the nose, and then in the mouth.

THE ORGAN OF SMELL.

With most people the nose is nothing more than that triangular and pyramidal projection situated in the middle of the face, between the eyes and mouth, without their doubting the least in the world, the beauty and delicacy of the texture which lines its exterior.

Perhaps it may not be inappropriate to remark, that we shall be well paid, for the labor that writing this appendix cost us, if, after having sketched this short anatomical picture, we should see some snuffers renounce their detestable habit, in just fear of what we shall be able to inspire them, of destroying one of the five senses which procures us the sweetest and most agreeable sensations, except, understand me, that of the powder which we are now combating.

The nostrils are the two cavities of the nose, hollowed out of the thickness of the face, which extend backward and terminate in other cavities called *frontal sinuses, &c.*

A mucous membrane, quite thick and always humid, in the tissue of which the olfactory nerves, as well as a great number of other nerves, and blood-vessels are spread, line their interior surface, and is prolonged in the sinuses which joins them, and covers the projections and depressions of their walls. This soft and spongy membrane, called *pituitary*, when healthy, secretes mucus.

We should have added, the eyes communicate with the nostrils by the aid of two canals which conduct in them, constantly, a part of the tears which have served to moisten the eyeballs.

We should not omit to state, that the nasal fossas, or nostrils, communicate by sympathy with the brain and stomach, &c.; and that they are the special seat of the sense of smell, the uses of which are to inform us immediately of the odoriferous particles suspended in the atmosphere, from which information two secondary properties are deduced, viz. :—

1st, To watch the qualities of the air ; and

2nd, To control the quality of certain aliments.

Indeed, one would suppose that the sense of smell procured man too many joys for him to make it a sport to abuse it.

Man derives great pleasure at first in smelling the enervating perfume which the chalice of sweet and beautiful flowers exhale; then, he happens, by degrees, to love the odor of certain emanations, which the dirtiest animal refuses to smell. A most astonishing creature is man!

All confirmed chewers are more or less subject to long standing diseases of the stomach and liver. I might cite here many cases to prove this fact from the writings of others, and from my own observation and experience, but I refrain, and deem it unnecessary to say more than that self-respect—respect for our relations and friends, and for strangers—should induce tobacco chewers to practise more decency in the consumption of the weed, and not spit here, there, and everywhere, irrespective of persons and places.

It is not agreeable to gentlemen chewers to be impolite in any other respect, except in the use of tobacco; and they do carry their impoliteness to extremes sometimes, and then expect people to bear it in silence. They are generally treated with silent contempt, and allowed to indulge their barbarous habits to their hearts' content. They only injure themselves, and sometimes the property of others; but, as they injure themselves more than the property of others, the owners of the latter, in the depths of their sympathy for the unfortunate authors of the injury, are generally polite enough to pass it over unnoticed. However, as we have many laws to correct nuisances, and as the use of tobacco is one of the greatest nuisances that stalks abroad, there should be laws enenacted, regulating it, and not allow men to make barbarians and beasts of themselves, to the great annoyance of decent people.

You often hear smokers and chewers remark how disgusting and filthy snuffing is ; and the knight of the snuffbox has an equal horror of the habit of smoking or chewing, and considers his habit as the gentleman's delight.

What *nonsensical contradictions* tobacco consumers are. They all admit, if put to the test, that it is a beastly, unhealthy, and filthy habit, and excuse themselves on the grounds that they used it to preserve their teeth, or to keep them from becoming too fleshy, or perhaps to kill them, and keep the blue devils away.

I hope these pages may convince all such persons that they labor under a great error, and that the weed will produce the very ills they wish to escape.

Gentlemen, votaries of the weed, think —
" If then tobacconing be good, how is't
That lewdest, loosest, basest, most foolish,
The most unthrifty, most intemperate,
Most vicious, most debauched, most desperate,
Pursue it most ? The WISEST and the BEST
Abhor it, shun it, flee it as the pest !"

The German physiologists affirm, that of twenty deaths of men between eighteen and twenty years of age in Germany, ten orginate in the waste of the constitution by smoking tobacco.

The great prevalence of consumption in the United States is due in part to the general and excessive use of tobacco.

A RAILROAD DREAM.

BY MRS. F. D. GAGE.

"Corrupting the air with noisome smells," is an actionable nuisance. See Blackstone, "Trespass," or "Private Wrongs."

Sitting in a rail-car, flying on by steam,
Head against the casement, dreamed a curious dream;
Yet I could not think it all a thing ideal,
For, though very monstrous, it was very real.

First there came a gentleman in his patent leather,
Collar, bosom, wristbands, overcoat for weather,
In the height of fashion, watch-key, hat and glove,
And, with air professional, — SPIT upon the stove.

Near him sat a parson, telling how the Lord
Sent the great revivals, blessed the preached word;
But my dream discovered he was not above
Honey-dew or fine-cut — spitting on the stove.

Next came a trader, pockets full of cash,
Talked about the country going all to smash;
" War and abolition did the thing, by Jove,"
Tipped his wicker-bottle — spit upon the stove.

Then a jolly farmer, bragging of his wheat,
Thought his hogs and horses no where could be beat;
" Like to sell his Durhams, by the head or drove,"
Kept his jaws a wagging — spit upon the stove.

Paddy thought 'twas " quare " like, to be sitting still,
All the whilst a goin', over bog and hill,
'Twas a glorious counthra, sure, as he could prove —
Equal to his betters — spitting on the stove.

Witless, perfumed dandy, putting on his air,
Flourished diamond breast-pin, smoked in forward car;
Talked about our army, " 'Twas too slow, by Jove,"
Twirled a carrot moustache — spit upon the stove.

Little boy in short-coat, wants to be a man,
Following example as the surest plan;
Watches gent and parson — copies every move,
And with Pat and trader — spits upon the stove.

Soon the flying rail-car reeks with nauseous steam;
Ladies almost fainting, children in a scream;
Husband asking lady: " What's the matter, love?
Have a glass of water?" — spits upon the stove.

On we go, still flying, not a breath of air
Fit for Christian people, in the crowded car;
Sickening, fainting, dying, ladies make a move,
Gent throws up the window — spits upon the stove.

Now, perchance this dreaming was not all a dream;
Think I've had a steaming travelling by steam;
'Tis a public nuisance, any one can prove,
" All the air corrupting — spitting on the stove."

Talk of ladies flounces, ribbons, jewels, flowers,
Crinolines and perfumes, gossip, idle hours;
Put all faults together, which men can't approve,
And they're not a match for — spitting on the stove.

Men *will* call us angels, wonder if they think
Such a nauseous vapor, *angel meat and drink?*
Wonder if they'll do so when they get " above?"
Below it *would be handier* — spitting on the stove.

CONSULTATION.

In treating pulmonary disease, a personal examination of the patient is desirable, but not absolutely essential. An intimate acquaintance with the symptoms which attend the various stages of the disease, enables the physician to determine with great accuracy, from a full and minute statement of any case, the condition of the patient, so as to enable him to prescribe adequately and with success. A letter replying to the questions which will be found on pages 214 to 219 of this volume, will meet with prompt attention.

We would earnestly advise the patient to consult us personally at our office, when convenient to do so. The facilities for a minute investigation and discrimination of every feature of the case are so much greater, that a perfect diagnosis, so requisite to form the basis of a successful treatment, is sure to be made. Our treatment is prepared, accordingly, in strict relation to the features of the case and the demands of the patient; and, what is still an important consideration in aiding the cure, the personal encouragement and favorable impression made upon the mind of the patient has a wonderful effect in arousing and supporting the energies of the nervous system, and elevating hope, which causes the medicinal remedies to do a double good. But patients at a distance, who cannot find it convenient, will do well to consult us by letter (which must always enclose a stamp), describing their case in every minute particular; as to cause, seat, local or general, constitutional or hereditary, degree of suffering, appetite, state of the bowels and digestive organs, and the complication with other organs, as the kidneys, or urinary complaints, or affections of the reproductive organs,—as these all have a sympathy of action, and must be treated to insure success.

QUESTIONS FOR INVALIDS.

As I have had the happiness of relieving very many consumptive and other invalids whom I have never seen, I subjoin a number of questions, of which the invalid, wishing to consult me by letter, will please answer such as may concern him, adding any further remarks that may be necessary to a clear description of his case. I can then give my advice almost as successfully as though the patient were himself present; still, if convenient, it is better that I should see him.

Address, DR. CHARLES R. BROADBENT, 99 Court Street, Boston.

TO INVALID LADIES.

What is your name, age, occupation, residence, so that a letter may reach you? Where born and brought up? Delicate or good constitution? Height? Slender or broad figure? Fleshy or lean? Erect or stooping? Chest full and straight, or contracted, flat and stooping? What is the color of your hair, eyes, and complexion? To what diseases are your family subject? Any died of Asthma, Scrofula, Heart Diseases, Dropsy, Cancer, or Consumption? Are you subject to Asthma or short breathing? Any humor, salt rheum, or skin diseases? Any head-ache, or pain in the chest, neck, spine, shoulders, back, stomach, bowels, sides, or limbs? Any sore throat, swelled tonsils, heat or dryness in the throat, weak voice, loss of voice, hoarseness, catarrh in head, nose, or throat? Any cough? How long had it? Do you cough up anything? How much? What kind, &c.? When cough most? When raise most? Ever raise blood? How many times? How much? On which side lay best, if either? On full breathing, do your ribs rise equally all over your chest, or do the ribs rise better on one side or part than another? Have you daily chills, or fever, or night-sweats? Are you confined to your bed or room, or the house, or do you go out daily? Any palpitation or distress at the heart, or stoppage of circulation? Are you nervous or paralytic, or have fits? Any bad dreams, and their effects? Any dyspepsia, sore stomach, or distress, or pressure at the stomach? After eating, does food rise? Ever sick stomach to vomit? Ever any sinking, exhausted, all-gone feeling at top of chest, pit of stomach, or sides, or bowels, or across you? Appetite good, bad, or capricious? Bowels regular, costive, or diarrhœa? Any external or bleeding or blind piles, or fistula, weak back, heat in your back or any part, hot flashes? Have a rupture? Suspect having worms? What kind? Any gravel or kidney complaints? Water stoppage, or free, or too much, scanty or scalding, or settlings? Cold or burning feet? Bloating anywhere? Much wind in stomach or bowels? Rheumatism or neuralgia? Any deformity? Ever any wounds? Long fevers? Took much medicine or mercury? Fever sores? Bilious habitually? Married or single, or widow? Had any children? Suffered miscarriages or floodings? Ever rise from bed feeling quite smart, but, on exercising, soon obliged to sit or lay down all exhausted, or discouraged with head-ache? Natural periods easy, painful, regular or irregular, or stopped? If so, how long, and why? In the family-way? Any bearing down or female complaints? What have you done for these complaints? Can you read aloud, or talk long, or walk well, or do little work, without usual fatigue? Are you in indigent or easy circumstances? Have you good teeth? Do you work hard, go out much, or reverse?

TO INVALID GENTLEMEN.

What is your name, occupation, or profession? Residence, so that a letter will reach you? Where born and brought up? Delicate or good constitution? Height? Slender or broad figure? Fleshy or lean? Person erect or stooping? Chest full and straight, or stooping and contracted? Constitution delicate or robust? What is the color of your hair, whiskers, eyes, and complexion? To what diseases are your family subject? Any died of Asthma, Scrofula, Heart Disease, or Consumption? Are you subject to Asthma or short breathing? Any humor, scrofula, salt rheum, or skin diseases? Any head-ache, or pain in the chest, neck, spine, shoulders, back, stomach, bowels, sides, or limbs? Any sore throat, swelled tonsils, heat or dryness in the throat, weak voice, loss of voice, hoarseness, catarrh in head, nose, or throat? Any cough? How long had it? Do you cough up anything? How much? What kind, &c.? When cough most? When raise most? Ever raise blood? How many times? How much? On which side lay best, if either? On full breathing, do your ribs rise equally all over your chest, or do the ribs rise better on one side or part than another? Have you daily chills, or fever, or night-sweats? short breathing or asthma? Are you confined to your bed or room, or the house, or do you go out daily? Any palpitation or distress at the heart, or stoppage of circulation? Are you nervous or paralytic, or have fits? Any bad dreams, and their effects? Any dyspepsia, sore stomach, or distress, or pressure at the stomach, after eating? or ever sick stomach to vomit, or food rise after eating? Ever any sinking, exhausted, all-gone feeling at top of chest, pit of stomach, or in the stomach or sides, or bowels, or across the bowels? Appetite good, bad, or capricious? Bowels regular, costive, or diarrhœa? Any external or bleeding or blind piles, weak back? Have a rupture? Suspect having worms? What kind? Any gravel or kidney complaints? Water stoppage, or free, settling, scanty, or scalding, or too much? Any heat in your back or any part? Cold or burning feet? Bloating anywhere? Much wind in stomach or bowels? Pains in your limbs? Rheumatism or neuralgia? Any deformity? Ever any wounds? Long fevers? Took much medicine or mercury? Fever sores? Bilious? Clear complexion? What done for these complaints? How long? Are you married or single? Can you read aloud, or talk long, or walk actively, or do work without unusual fatigue? In indigent or easy circumstances? Do you work hard, or take active exercise, or the reverse? Dropsy or cancers? Have you good teeth?

Hundreds of cases are successfully treated every year abroad that are never seen by Dr. Broadbent, so perfect is this system of treatment.

Dr. Broadbent has, between March, 1847, and the corresponding month of 1857, delivered nine hundred lectures to large audiences, on Physiology, Health, &c., in all the principal cities and large towns of New England, and has, in the same time, been consulted by fifteen or twenty thousand invalids of all descriptions.

IMPORTANT TESTIMONY FROM PATIENTS.

―

Chelsea, Sept. 15, 1858.

Dr. C. R. Broadbent,

Dear Sir: — I am aware how little importance is usually attached to the various advertisements and certificates of cures which make their appearance in the newspapers of the day, and yet I feel that it is but an act of justice to you, as well as to the multitude suffering from pulmonary diseases which have heretofore been regarded incurable, that I should make a simple statement of my own case, and the benefit I have received from your mode of treatment.

Six months ago I had every symptom of confirmed and deep-seated consumption — a severe cough, chills and fever, with cold night-sweats, and daily expectoration of thick heavy matter. For months I had not known the pleasure of a comfortable night's rest. I availed myself of the best medical advice, and was under the care of several very respectable physicians, but with no lasting beneficial results.

At length a neighbor of mine, who had been cured

under your treatment, urged me to consult you, and finally lent me your pamphlet on Inhalation. From a careful perusal of its contents, I became fully convinced that Inhalation was my only hope, and resolved at once to give it a thorough and faithful trial.

I called upon you about the 15th of last March, and, after you had made a careful examination of my case, you encouraged me to hope, and thought you might be able to cure me.

From the daily use of your inhalants, I soon found sensible relief. My rest, which had been disturbed and broken, now became easy, and, in a word, I could sleep comfortably all night. My spells of coughing were less frequent, the expectoration gradually diminished, I gained in flesh and strength, and, at the present time, regard myself perfectly cured, being able to endure as much hardship as ever I could.

I have made this statement of my case more to encourage others, similarly afflicted, to hope for relief, knowing that your practice is too well established to require any additional testimony from me.

Very respectfully yours,

MRS. MOSES A. ILSLEY.

West Roxbury, Oct. 15, 1861.

DR. C. R. BROADBENT,

Dear Sir: — I called at your office last spring, stated my case, ascertained your mode of treatment, and so entirely convinced did I feel that this was the long sought remedy which was to restore me to health, that I resolved to commence at once. I used your Inhalents every morning and evening, the effect seemed truly wonderful. The soreness gradually left my lungs; the expectoration, which was very copious and purulent, diminished from day to day, while the irritation in my lungs and throat entirely subsided. I now discontinued the use of the inhaler, except at intervals, when I felt any slight return of the irritation in my throat. By strictly following your directions, the soreness and inflammation of my lungs rapidly disappeared, and I once more lie down and sleep comfortably all night, and seldom feel any inclination to cough. By your advice, I keep your remedies constantly on hand, and whenever I feel any irritation in my throat, I immediately seek the magic inhaler, and soon find myself all right again.

I feel under deep obligations to you, sir, for the relief I have obtained both in body and mind, and you may be assured that I shall do all in my power to repay you, in some measure, for your kindness and attention to me, by inducing all who are afflicted with pulmonary affections to seek what I believe to be the most sure and effectualy means on earth for the cure of this most fatal disease.

Yours, very truly,

MISS EMILY A. LANG.

Remarks. — I will add, by way of explanation, that the above cases were unmistakable, genuine Tubercular Consumption, in a somewhat advanced state. Their disease was pronounced hopeless, and all further means for their recovery, by physicians and friends, had been abandoned. Under these circumstances, I had but little confidence that anything beyond mere temporary relief could be hoped for. The results stand out in bold relief, and I can but feel that the perfect success with which the treatment of these important cases has been attended, affords us great encouragement in the future management of this formidable malady.

This case was nearly as bad as the last two, and her husband writes as follows:—

Natick, Mass., Jan. 20, 1862.

Dr. BROADBENT,

Dear Sir: — Will you please send my wife one bottle more, each, of the Electrical Medicine, and one of the Sanative. She thinks she ought to take one bottle more of each kind, to feel perfectly well again; and that will be, I think, all the medicine she will require.

I think you have saved my wife from an early grave, for which I shall be your grateful friend.

Yours truly,

JOHN CARTER.

This lady was only under my treatment about three months before she got well.

I could fill a book much larger that this, with similar letters to the above, which I have received from different patients during the past eighteen years; but for want of space in this little book, I will give only the *names* and *residences* of the persons who have received my medical treatment, and who have been *cured* by the same.

Any person who disbelieves the correctness or truth of my statements can satisfy him or herself, by writing to, or calling on, any of the following persons:—

William R. Swan,	117 Central Ave., Chelsea, Mass.
Miss M. A. Edwards,	" "
Mr. Augustus Beneford,	" "
Mrs. E. A. Cobb,	" "
Mr. John Walter, Commission Merchant, (heart disease),	Head of Long Wharf, Boston.
Mr. Albert Patch,	Waltham, Mass.
Mr. Benjamin F. Brown,	" "
Mrs. A. W. Darling,	Exeter, N. H.
Mrs. Charles A. Marsh,	Medford, Mass.
Miss Merriam Glidden,	Dorchester, "
Mrs. Cynthia Chevalier,	Charleston, "
Miss Jennett Dickie,	W. Cambridge, "
Mr. Isaac Gale,	Natick, "
Mrs. Cornelious L. White,	Randolph, "
Mr. Elijah E. Lummus, Postmaster,	N. Beverly, "

Mr. Nathaniel S. Gould,	Wenham, Mass.
" C. G. Otis,	Bath, Maine.
" T. P. Brown,	Wenham, Mass.
" and Mrs. Henry Parkhurst,	Roxbury, Mass.
" and Mrs. John J. Merrill,	" "
" Beckworth,	Natick, "
Mrs. Benjamin O. Hibbard,	S. Boston, "
" Robert Humphrey,	Webster, "
" L. S. Chandler, 30 Austin St., Charlestown, "
" Joseph W. Delano,	Boston, "
Miss A. Maria Bunker,	" "
Mr. E. P. Palmer,	Gardner, Maine.
Mrs. Ephraim B. Lewis,	Lowell, Mass.
" M. W. Manning,	Springfield, "
" Harvey D. Chapin,	" "
" M. Prentice,	Pittsfield, "
" Mary A. Vibert,	" "
Mr. J. W. Darby,	" "
Mrs. Wm. H. Bowman,	Albany, N. Y.
" J. S. Clark,	" "
Mr. Edward James,	" "
Mrs. Joshua A. Rich,	Harwich, Mass.
" G. W. Lang,	Boston, "
" Mrs. Susan Junio,	Charlestown, "
" Horace Walker,	Medford, "

I will not weary your patience by giving any more names. The above, with thousands of others, I have, with the blessing of Providence, been instrumental in restoring to pretty good health and strength by my mode of treatment.

CONTENTS.

INDEX TO SUBJECTS.

Introduction..Page 5
Consumption; its Cause and Curability,........................ 9
Symptoms of Consumption,...................................... 20
Practical Observations on the Causes and Curability of Tubercular and Bronchial Consumption,............................. 27
Consumption, and its different varieties,...................... 33
Hemorrage, or Bleeding of the Lungs,.......................... 40
Asthma; Causes, Symptoms, and Treatment by Medicated Inhalation, 45
" its Treatment,... 47
Consumption; Cause, Symptoms, Prevention and Specific Treatment, 50
" its Symptoms,................................... 66
Bronchitis; Ministers' Sore Throat,............................ 71
Laryngitis; Clergyman's Sore Throat,.......................... 73
Bronchial Consumption,.. 75
Pleuretic Consumption,.. 77
Dyspeptic Consumption,.. 80
Coughs and Colds,... 82
Consumption; A New and Accurate Method for the Diagnosis of... 86
An inquiry concerning the nature of Disease, and a Rational Mode of Cure,... 96
General Debility,...100
The Skin and its Offices,.....................................105

INDEX.

Diet, ... 108
Varicose Veins and Humors, ... 109
Hemorrhoids, or Piles, ... 111
Costiveness; Manner of Curing, ... 114
Chronic Diseases, especially the Nervous Diseases of Women, ... 118
Epilepsy, or Fits, ... 121
The Stomach, ... 133
The Heart, ... 138
Tight Lacing, ... 143
Gravel, produced by Falling of the Bowels, &c. 145
Air and Ventilation, ... 147
Sleep, ... 151
Dyspepsia, ... 155
Erysipelas, ... 160
Dropsy, ... 164
Spinal Diseases; Pain in the Side; Beds, and Lying in Beds, ... 166
Climate, ... 168
Treatment of Diseases of the Lungs and Air-Passages, by the Inhalation of Cold and Warm Medicated Vapors, ... 169
Inhalants, what made of, ... 172
Conclusion, ... 173
Phrenology, ... 175
Mesmerism, ... 181
Tobacco: its action on the Health, and its influence on the Morals and Intelligence of Man, ... 187
    The organic changes which Tobacco produces in the nose, 199
    A Railroad Dream, (*Gage,*) 209
Consultation, ... 212
Questions for Invalids, ... 214
Important Testimony from Patients, ... 219

INDEX TO ENGRAVINGS.

The Whole System,........ ....Opposite title.
Back View of a Skeleton,................................Page 8
The Air-Passages of the Right and Left Lung,.................. 33
The Right Lung and Air-Passsages of the Left Lung,............. 50
The Human Form—Healthy and Dropsical,....................104
Scrofulous Humor,...109
Sole Leg,...110
The Nervous System—View of the Brain and Nerves,...........117
The Brain,..121
The Internal Organs,..132
The Heart and its Blood Vessels,.............................138
Tight Lacing, &c.,..143
Kidneys, Ureters, &c.,......................................144
Inhalation, ...169
Phrenological Cut,..175

DR. BROADBENT'S MEDICINES.

PREPARED ONLY BY HIMSELF.

DR. BROADBENT'S
Medicated Inhaling Balm Vapor.

For curing Laryngitis, Acute and Chronic Catarrh of the Air-Passages, Bronchial and Tubercular Consumption.

This preparation is one of the most certain agents ever yet discovered, for soothing, mitigating and curing inflamed surfaces, Cough, Hoarseness, Loss of Voice, Asthma, Difficulty of Breathing, Shortness of Breath, Pain in the Lungs and Chest. It readily enters every minute part of the lungs, the air-tubes and cells; reduces large bronchial glands, stimulating ulcerated surfaces to a healthy and healing action; dissolves tubercles, which press upon the blood-vessels, and cause bleeding; and causes the absorbents to take out tubercular deposits from the lungs.

DIRECTIONS. — Put from one to three teaspoonfuls of this Balm into a cup half full of warm water; then inhale the steam from five to twenty minutes at a time, every night and morning, from an inhaler.

BOSTON LUNG INSTITUTE, Boston, Mass.

DR. C. R. BROADBENT'S
EXPECTORANT INHALANT.

This Vapor is to be used with the BALM, at such times as the Lungs are confined, or when it is hard to expectorate the matter or mucus from the Lungs. It greatly loosens or thins the matter secreted, and enables the patient to expectorate, or raise it up, with greater facility, and freedom, without the coughing or rasping effort, which, if allowed, would irritate the lungs, and exhaust the patient.

DIRECTIONS. — One teaspoonful or more is to be mixed with Balm Vapor, and inhaled, as usual. In severe cases of STUFFING, or confined state of the air-passages, use it freely; and in all sudden attacks of *Asthma* it can be used in large doses until relief is obtained.

N. B. — Shake the bottle well from the bottom.

Dr. Broadbent's Embrocation.

This Embrocation affords immediate and certain relief for all pains and aches and soreness, either acute, chronic or dull; pleuretic pains; rheumatic, neuralgic, or spasmodic, — either in the chest, side, joints, back, head, or any part of the body.

DIRECTIONS. — Saturate a small piece of flannel cloth with the Embrocation, using from a teaspoonful to a tablespoonful, according to the emergency of the pain or disease to be overcome; then rub the part smartly from five to fifteen minutes every night, and oftener if required.

DR. BROADBENT'S
ANTI-BILIOUS POWDERS.

These Powders are mild, yet efficient, and occasion no sickness, pain, or uneasiness. They have one most important quality, not found in any other cathartic in use, viz: *they do not leave the bowels weakened or costive, and may be used any length of time without loosing their efficiency.*

They have tonic properties, which strengthen the stomach and sustain the vigor of the system while a cathartic effect is being produced. In all cases of habitual costiveness, too full a habit, palpitation of the heart, indigestion, torpid liver, pressure in the head, wind in the stomach or bowels, biliousness, jaundice, all impurities of the blood, skin disease, salt rheum, spots on the face, and whenever a cathartic is desired, these powders are so compounded as to meet the exigency. The most delicate may take them without being weakened or made sick, and upon the most robust, by increasing the dose, they act with efficiency. No family once using these powders will ever abandon them for any other.

DIRECTIONS.— Take one of these Powders every other week, as follows, viz: Put one of them into a cupful of hot water, sweeten it, and let it stand until cold before you drink it; then drink, grounds and all.

DR. BROADBENT'S
Sanative for Kidney and Urinary Diseases.

The Sanative is a sure and permanent remedy for Gravel and Stone, Inflammations of the Bladder and Kidney, Scalding or Burning heat of the Water, Diabetes, Offensive condition of the Urine, Difficulty of Urinating, and inability to retain the water in consequence of relaxation and debility. Ulcerations of the Bladder; Morbid Discharges indicated by deposits of sediments and phosphates in the water; Cancers and Fatty Degenerations; and Bright's Disease of the Kidney; and Dropsical Effusion in any part of the body,— are all cured by a proper use of this Sanative.

DIRECTIONS.— One teaspoonful is to be taken three times a day.

Dr. Broadbent's Heart Sanative.

This will be confessed, by all who may make a trial of it, a most magical remedy in all cases of palpitation of the heart, or any form of heart disease. This complaint is usually considered a very dangerous and fatal one, and, unless properly treated, it is so. It is, at all events, a most distressing one.

This Sanative, in cases of heart difficulty, gives the most delightful relief, soothes and calms the throbbings of the heart, tranquilizes the arterial excitement, and equalizes the circulation. In recent cases no other remedy is needed to CURE.

DIRECTIONS.— One teaspoonful to be taken every night and morning.

DR. C. R. BROADBENT'S
TWO ELECTRICAL MEDICINES.

For disturbed bilious action—torpid, congested, or otherwise deranged liver—for all forms of biliousness—for headache of any kind, costiveness, sick stomach, flatulence, diarrhœa, indigestion, piles, determination of blood to the head, and for malarial fevers, &c., this medicine is a specific, quite doing away with the use of calomel, possessing as it does the alterative and useful, without any of the hurtful properties of that drug.

DIRECTIONS.— Take one teaspoonful of these every morning and night.

DR. BROADBENT'S
Medicine for Nervous Debility.

This is a truly happy and fortunate preparation, combining the concentrated active principles of a recently discovered nervine; its action upon the prostrated energies of the nervous system is wonderful, and it will cure every kind of nervous debility.

DIRECTIONS.— Take one teaspoonful of this every night when you go to bed.

Price from two to three dollars per bottle for any of these medicines, according to size; and one dollar extra for the Inhaler. Sent to any person safely by Express.

www.ingramcontent.com/pod-product-compliance
Lightning Source LLC
Chambersburg PA
CBHW021828230426
43669CB00008B/897